Here For The D
A Maternity Care Guide Bringing Humor and Empowerment to the Delivery, Decisions and the Other D

Dev Honey, CPM, LM

Here For The D
*A Maternity Care Guide Bringing Humor and Empowerment to the Delivery,
Decisions and the Other D*

Published by Birds and Bees Midwifery LLC
Smithfield, VA
www.devhoneybooks.com
Copyright 2023 by Melissa Honey
ISBN 979-8-9874902-0-4 (paperback)
ISBN 979-8-9874902-1-1 (epub)

Cover photo by Whitney Popp, Popp Photography

Author photo by Jessica Rinehart, The Heart of Now Photography

Makeup by Noelle Cahoon with Blush757

Editor Dawn Brotherton, Blue Dragon Publishing, LLC

I think it's only appropriate to dedicate this to moms. They are, after all, the reason for this book. To moms everywhere, you are warriors, and I am so proud of you.

Particularly my mom. I know you wanted me to be ladylike, but I decided to be everything else. I love you.

Table of Contents

Introduction

I'm a working mom with a partner, a family, a social life, religious convictions and a workout plan, who is just trying to stay hydrated and keep her nails fabulous!

Throughout my career, I have found myself recommending a stack of books to pregnant women. This book came out of my desire to sum it up, reduce the overwhelm and remind moms that they got this. You do not have to be a pregnancy expert to be pregnant, or a psychology expert to be a good mom. I try to keep it simple and down to the need-to-know—even though sometimes I include random information or stories just for emphasis and fun. If you want to know more, I encourage you to explore that desire but don't feel pressured to. A little knowledge, a good care provider, and your intuition are enough.

In running a family, we often feel like we have to know and be everything. We are the financial planner, the chef, the teacher, the therapist, the chauffeur, the mechanic, the housekeeper, the appliance repair person, not to mention all the roles we play for our partners, our jobs, our extended family, our pets and our communities. Pause here, take a deep breath, one . . . two . . . three . . . You are amazing, and worthy and enough exactly how you are now. Without investing, without being the ultimate play-date mom, without reading that stack of books or even this book, without having the newest car, without makeup, without your hair done, without losing the weight or gaining the weight, without following the majority, without upgrading any part of your life or yourself, you are enough **right now**. You decide what you do with your time, and that is enough of a reason to do anything.

In this book I talk a lot about midwifery care and home birth, because that's my wheelhouse, but this information is relevant no matter which care provider you use a hospital-based midwife, OB-GYN or no pregnancy care at all. While I recommend having a care provider during pregnancy and birth—even the hands-off kind—I encourage all moms to make the choice that feels best for them, not the fear-based choice but the loving, deeply resonating choice.

Home birth is an option for many moms. When natural birth is safe, people should always feel like they have the ability to choose how and where to birth. If your choice is a hospital or epidural because that is what feels right for you, then that is ideal for you. If circumstances have arisen that make a C-section necessary (history of a C-section does not always make a second C-section necessary, by the way), then you should still feel heard, respected and cared for in that moment.

We, as humans, should be allowed to choose without judgment or fear mongering. My hope for the future is that we open up the discussion and share information in a loving way that allows for our growth. Pregnancy, labor and birth are such personal, monumental experiences, why not make it your own? Why not make all the choices? Be informed, be deeply moved, be in tune with your body and trust what you know. In the words of Nelson Mandela, "May your choices reflect your hopes not your fears."

In this book, I try to be all-inclusive and not make any preconceived judgment on the many ways to get pregnant, experience pregnancy and birth, create families, experience/express gender, or any individual's sexual orientation, religious beliefs, mental health, personal backgrounds, pronouns, relationship status or ethnicity. I am a middle-class, Jewish, white woman, so please excuse any unintentional ignorance in the language I use; I try my best.

I refer to the person who is pregnant as the "mom" and the "woman" often throughout this book; however, I acknowledge those individuals that can get pregnant but identify as him/he or them/

they. I see you. Your pregnancies are just as valid and just as stunning as anyone's. Curing the world of hate is outside the realm of this book but maybe it's a step toward making the world a little better by adding some love, respect and power to the lives of a pregnant person and their families. This book goes out to all those who experience pregnancy and birth, regardless of race, gender, religion, socioeconomic status, age or any other thing that makes us different from one another. It is always in my heart that we can come together as humans and work to repair our brokenness.

You may notice that I use the spelling G-d for the name of a higher power. This is a Jewish practice to prevent desecrating the name. While some sects of Judaism believe the ordinance to not desecrate The Name only applies when it is written in Hebrew, I'd rather not take any chances. When deciding whether to honor my religious beliefs or spell out the name, I felt better leaving the dash. You can apply your own meaning to the name of G-d, no matter how it looks.

Lastly, this book contains what might be considered explicit language. I am a student of languages and so value the importance of the impact of the human language. Pregnancy and birth are just too deep, too big for everyday words; sometimes I need to swear. If this language offends you, hopefully you can get passed it and absorb the information and overall message. If you can't, this book may not be for you, and that's okay.

I have two goals for this book. The first is to empower and inform pregnant people. The second is to stir up a discussion about maternity care in the United States. There is room for growth in both these areas, and it will only happen at the hands of people willing to explore their options and confidently choose.

With love, hope, grace and a sense of humor, I offer you—with a D for Delivery, Discussion and the other D word—*Here For The D*.

Chapter One

Let's Do This Thing

G-d is good. G-d, protect me and hold me. Thaaaank you, G-d. Praise G-d," she said softly between contractions.

I watched as her belly began to change shape, indicating the contraction was starting.

"TRUCK! Truck of shiiiiiiit! Holy truck of my mother! CROUTONS!"

She let out a long breath when the contraction let go. "G-d is good, praise G-d."

And on and on she went, praising G-d and cursing croutons until her baby was tucked warmly in her arms. She took her gaze off her sweet bundle for a moment to look at me and say, "Birth is nuts."

I couldn't agree more, we are part of this wild, spectacular thing that is completely nuts.

Welcome to motherhood/parenthood. You love your child(ren) with immense, unconditional love, and you are so happy when they go to bed. The focus of this book is you, the badass, boundary-setting, empowered, emotionally raw, deep feeling, flowing and pregnant you. Since you're reading this, I assume you're pregnant, were pregnant or you are trying to be pregnant. No matter which of those applies, pause here and celebrate. You are amazing. Amazing just for taking this journey! I know, I know. You might not feel

11

amazing, certainly not all the time, but you are ALL the time. You were just made that way.

Ready for the tough love part? It's time to take a look at yourself, not a mean, over-critical look but an honest, loving look. Turn inward and look at yourself as if you are your own child. You are five years old in your pajamas carrying a bowl of cereal and spilling some milk with every step. You sit down at the table across from your adult self and say, "We've been negative. We've been complaining. We've been worrying. Oh my, have we been worrying! We've been doubting ourselves. We've been feeling worthless. We've been fearful. We've lacked accountability, and even in moments where we've admitted to what we are doing wrong, we lack the discipline to do something about it, but that's done now."

Now say to your younger self, "There is no reason to worry, no reason to doubt, no reason to fear, because I trust myself. I know I am worthy. I know I have faced many difficult things in the past, and I have always been okay; I have always gotten through. I can do it again. I can make anything happen. I can do it better. I am strong, capable, fearless, believing and worthy."

Good, now we can do this.

The first thing I ask of my clients is self-awareness, accountability and discipline. Don't be afraid to examine yourself and your life. Do you know yourself? Do you trust yourself? Are you living the life that feels best for you? Are you treating people well? Do you have an attitude of gratitude? Are you addressing your insecurities, your fears, your shortcomings, your trauma responses and your limiting beliefs? Hold yourself up to the light and take a look. Look with love, not shame, and strive for something better.

I add discipline, even though we are raised to believe that's a negative word, because it's one thing to say "I have this bad habit." It's another thing to get up and do something about it. Self-discipline creates real change, real improvement and real long-term benefits. Self-discipline is an act of self-love.

I have to admit I really like that my bachelor's of science degree is abbreviated as BS, because, yes, I have a degree in BS, and I can tell when my clients are full of it. It's time for you to own up to your bullshit. I mean genuine accountability, the stuff that cuts you deep. Being truly in love with ourselves means meeting the parts of us that are not yet parts we're proud of and moving toward improvement. This is your life, and no one is coming to do the work for you.

Okay, you've looked inward; you've pulled out your unflattering behavior and decided you are a grown, kind, loving, brave, generous and prosperous woman, and you have some things to slay. Throughout this book, I hope to help with some of the many choices you will make as you form into a mom, for the first or fifteenth time. If you have a care provider who does not give you choices—like real, informed, unbiased, non-fear-based choices—then fight for yourself. If that's not the care provider for you, keep on steppin'.

Your midwife is not there to tell you what you should do. Your midwife is a guide, there to explain the research to the best of her knowledge, share experiences, encourage you and let you know when something requires a little extra oomph. Your midwife is human and doesn't know everything, so there may be times when an additional provider or specialist becomes an important part of your team.

Fear should not dictate your decisions. Fear is a tool used to protect us from lions and motivate us to action before we die. Before you make any choice, sit back and ask yourself, are you making this decision from a place of fear, guilt or shame? You're better than that! Let's promise each other right now to make decisions from a strong, informed, deep-knowing, loving place. Sit all the way back, like to the back of your brain, and watch yourself make this decision. Don't judge, just watch what feelings come up for you. Honor those feelings, respect that part of yourself that wants to keep you safe, thank it for coming and then rise to the call that is truly best for you.

Research and scientific progress are not linear or definitive. One minute, researchers think they've developed a revolutionary medication to prevent miscarriage; the next minute, it actually caused cancer on a big scale. Studying pregnant women is difficult because the subject pool is small and widely varied. The research takes years and many reviews, only to be disproven decades later. I try to avoid absolute statements like "you will have this outcome." We can't predict the future; we can only calculate risk to the best of our ability and continue to learn. Historically it has taken about thirty years for policies in the field of obstetrics to change. This means that some are outdated, unnecessary or even dangerous policies, some are blanket policies that should actually only be applied to certain individuals, and some are valid, safe, necessary policies that have stood the test of time. Knowing which is which is difficult. In the end, we do our best, accept what we can't control and move forward. Your care provider should explain the risks and the benefits, then respect your decision, under the condition that it is not life threatening based on probability from valid studies, or illegal.

Often in maternity care, there is "routine care," which is what is expected for every pregnant person to do. Some examples of routine care include:

- Pee in a cup at every appointment (which, in your third trimester, should get every mom a trophy)
- Get an ultrasound at twenty weeks
- Get lab work done
- Get a Tdap vaccine
- Be tested for gestational diabetes by drinking a glucose mixture
- GBS swabs
- Birth laying on your back

Routine care is just code for "how we've done it for the last few decades or more." It's sometimes outdated, often dictated by insurance companies and puts providers on autopilot. However, having a routine-care checklist helps care providers be thorough, catch some conditions before they are a major problem and treat every client the same regardless of race, gender, religion etc.

As a type-A Sagittarius, I love a good checklist myself, but routine care should be evidence based and flexible because, Sweetheart, there is nothing routine about you. Do you have any specific concerns you want to address? Do you have any risk factors in yourself, your partner or either of your families that would factor into an assessment and make certain measures of care valuable? It's important to look at the whole picture as best we can. No intervention or procedure is completely risk free, even things done routinely. But declining intervention is also not without risk. These decisions are deeply personal and only for you to make.

All summed up, you're an individual, you can be trusted, you deserve good attentive care that is respectful and thorough and you can control your thoughts and actions. You are in charge of your life, Mama! Your care can and should be customized, which may mean foregoing some routine tasks, sticking to other parts of the routine and making additions.

What about when things suck? Pregnancy is not all "eating for two" and "you're glowing" (it's sweat, okay, I'm schvitzing like it's August in Arizona). There can be a lot of uncomfortable things during pregnancy. Not to mention the mental stress like "how will we afford it? Who will watch the baby while I'm at work, so I can afford to pay the sitter for watching the baby while I'm at work?"

Stop, breathe. Step fully into your power and know this: anything and everything only means what you make it mean. Read that again. Anything and everything only means what you make it mean. When we're babies, we don't know to call this person "mom." She has no label, no verbal cue; she just feels good. Only after the world around us assigns labels and meaning to things do we start to experience and assign meaning. The labels might get mixed up every now and then. Like when our parents exhibit an unhealthy behavior or pattern, and we translate that as love and carry it into our adult relationships.

Remember when you were a little kid and you found a stray animal? Your dad said, "Don't name it. You'll get attached."

In today's world, the typical advice is to label your feelings and share them with others. I would argue that particular strategy is for others, not for you. Sure, other people need the feeling identified so they can fabricate a way to help, but that feeling belongs to you, and if you name it, you'll get attached. Ever notice yourself saying, "I'm just so angry all the time"?

You have identified your outbursts at your partner or the kids as anger. You are not attached to this label. You've put it in the angry box, painted flames on the side and now decided that any and all manner of dealing with it will be based on that feeling being anger.

What if we didn't name it anger? What if we named it insecurity? A learned response from my past that I'm making excuses for? Low blood sugar? A hormone imbalance? My dissatisfaction with the choices I've made and need to blame someone else, because I can't handle being wrong?

Or what if you don't name it at all? It's nothing to you; it's not part of you or who you are. You can give it a new meaning, a new name, and change it completely, because you're disciplined AF remember? Everything is nothing until we name it.

Chapter Two

D is for. . .

Let's talk about sex (baby). You didn't think I was going to talk about pregnancy and skip over the fun part, did you? Let's get this out of the way right now. We all have an opinion about sex and what it should be. We all have a vision of the perfect sex life: every day, once a month, monogamous, polyamorous, threesome, anal, wait-for-marriage, leather, ropes, missionary, eyes closed, lights on, fifty shades, only for making babies, only for fun, toys, clit, g-spot, fingers, tongues, teeth, boobs and so many more words!

This is not a book about how you have sex or who you have sex with. This is about having sex in general and living in your body. No matter what the ideal sex situation is to you, sex is a vehicle for connection, power and bringing our vibration higher.

Many people think that the midwife steps in after conception has already happened, but truly, we talk about and counsel on sex more than you might think. Your body, your mood and your decision making are all controlled by your hormones. Midwives love to study hormones, and we want to know how yours are doing in many areas of your life. Share with your care provider when you notice changes in mood, sex drive, hair, skin, weight, nail beds and rational thinking that can't be traced back to an explainable factor in your life; it's all part of the puzzle that is your hormone health.

Most of us, at some point during our teenage years, got those weird stirs of desire and most of us had no idea what to do. Go easy on your parents; they didn't know how to talk about it. There's a lot of fear that talking about sex with teenagers will make them want to do it. This practice translates to teens who grow into adults who also don't talk about sex, or even worse, who feel shame for talking about sex, which contributes to a major lack of communication in relationships. Some people feel shame for even thinking about sex or for thinking about sex outside of the basics of the penis and vagina, especially for thoughts of sex outside the confines of marriage.

Maybe you were left to figure it out for yourself. The influences of television, school, media and social pressures put together a picture of sex that is not serving you anymore. Maybe you were taught that sex is currency. If you presented yourself as a sexually available being, flirted or performed favors, you got the attention you craved. You got invited into social circles; maybe he bought you lunch too.

Does sex = love? It's okay if this is what you believe; you were brought up in a system that understood sex a certain way. Your parents wanted what was best for you, but they were brought up in that system too, and they didn't know how to give you anything different. Forgive yourself. Forgive them.

Ask yourself and your partner what a healthy sex life looks like for you now. How often do you talk about sex? What are some new things you'd like to try? What are some things you don't actually like, or you wish would happen less often? What has sex meant to you in the past? What do you want it to mean now?

Start new, right now. Take off your clothes, stand in the mirror and say, "Thank you." Thank your body for being yours. Thank it for carrying you through heartache and triumphs. Thank your body for walking with you. Admire the strength that holds you upright, bask in the miracle that every cell in your body is working to keep you alive. Every cell loves you; every cell works in your favor. If any negative thoughts come up, tell that voice, "No thank you." You are here for love and gratitude.

How's your masturbation game? No really, when was the last time you enjoyed yourself? Have you ever? Do you regularly? Have you tried new things with yourself? Do you feel shame if you touch yourself? I understand you don't have to enjoy sex to make a baby, and self-pleasure is not required to make a baby either. If a baby is the only goal, then this chapter is about as useful as a knitted condom. If a baby isn't the only goal, your health and overall joy of life should be the goals.

This all starts with self-exploration. You are the first sexual being you'll meet. How are you going to introduce someone to your body when you haven't properly met it yourself? This is empowerment at its finest. In knowing your body, you also learn that you hold the keys to it. No one touches it without your permission, not even your doctor, your midwife or your partner. In loving and appreciating our bodies, we find eating healthy and engaging in physical activity as part of embracing the full potential of our bodies. This is where we find ecstasy, giving ourselves all kinds of physical pleasure without shame.

People who engage in self-pleasure are more in tune with their bodies. During pregnancy, this internal self-awareness is why midwives trust a mother's instinct. I'm not saying you must masturbate to have good intuition, but if you were looking for a reason . . . if you feel disconnected from your body or if you have extra anxiety around birthing that you can't seem to find the source of, maybe it's time you meet your body and show her how sexy she is.

While I encourage self-pleasure and self-exploration, I also recognize when this practice can go too far and damage relationships. If you or your partner can only orgasm through self-pleasure, would rather self-pleasure than connect to another during intercourse or if a porn addiction exists, these can be major struggles for relationships. I'm not the expert nor is this the book to solve porn addiction or lack of orgasm with a partner, but this is the book to encourage you to express gratitude for your partner's many wonderful qualities and know in your heart that you are an incredible person who can do hard things (didn't mean for that to be a sex pun, but sometimes the brilliance just flows from me).

Can we just talk about orgasms? Yes? Pour the tea, settle in. You probably already know the benefits of orgasms, the calorie burning, the happy hormones, the connection, the feel-good and the stress reduction. What I want to talk about is the how and why this might change during your pregnancy, including postpartum.

First, what is an orgasm? It always surprises me how many people don't know the textbook definition. It's muscle spasms. Now, don't get all offended by the simplicity of it; these are special muscle spasms that include ejaculation. This can also include your entire pelvic floor, your abs, glutes, thighs, legs, arms and face.

"Dev, I've never had a face-gasm. Am I okay?"

Yes, of course. Every human is different, and each orgasm can be different.

We are all wired differently. Throughout the body, a multitude of nerve endings detect pressure and determine pleasure feelings. These nerve endings are not in the same place in every person! Add the anatomy you were born with to your past experiences and you get your pleasure preferences for foreplay and orgasm. So, as your friend brags about her sensitive g-spot, don't start thinking something is wrong with you or whatever you're putting in there.

What feels good to us is not just personal preferences, it's in your anatomy. You don't have to orgasm or achieve orgasm the same way other people do, because you are uniquely built to orgasm in your own special way. This is why treating every new partner as though they are a completely different person is so important. They are! What gives them pleasure is not the same as your previous partner(s) (or it is because you have a type, Darling. We'll unpack that another time).

Begin with self-pleasure to learn what areas feel the most sensitive and stimulating to you. Next, gather information about yourself with each sexual experience then share these discoveries with the new person you're sleeping with. If you have waited until meeting the one, and you don't have any other sexual experiences to go off of, then fully embrace this opportunity to explore uncharted territory together. My hope is that this sharing is met with welcoming enthusiasm and an eagerness to please you and not with shame or judgement.

To be clear, I'm not referring to harmful fetishes or anything that might land you in jail. As you ease into a safe space where you can ask for the things that bring you pleasure, a whole glorious discovery of mutual pleasure, connection and orgasms is opened to you. Then you make a baby.

If a baby is the only goal of sex, you're missing out on an incredible opportunity for connection and a better pick-me-up than an energy drink. Start from the perspective of a midwife: good sex and birth are intertwined. After all, sex and birthing use the same parts and the same main hormone: oxytocin. Not only does sex produce oxytocin, making you happier and less stressed, but it also teaches your brain to acknowledge, control and embrace the sensations of the muscles in your pelvic floor. Recognizing these feelings and teaching your brain to relax these muscles makes childbirth less impeded by tight muscles and increases your sense of security in the moment of birth.

"Will I poke the baby?" This is the most frequently asked question from guys regarding sex during pregnancy. Sex during normal pregnancy is perfectly safe and recommended. Sex produces happy hormones that make you feel good and increase partner bonding. Dopamine and oxytocin are the main "feel good" hormones generated by sexual activity, including self-pleasure and sex with a partner(s). Sex feels good, and if it doesn't, sharing what doesn't feel good with your partner should only serve to deepen your intimate connection.

Have you ever read 1984? 1984 by George Orwell is a fiction novel about a government that takes over a society to the point of even policing peoples' thoughts. In the book, two people rebel against the government by . . . having sex. In that intimate moment of consensual nakedness, we are powerful AF! The act of sex scares governments, religious orders and parents all over the world. It's freedom, rebellion, power and pure self-indulgence. We can manifest during sex; we can connect deeply to the universe, G-d and whatever you believe in. Sex is awesome.

There are situations when it's recommended to avoid sex or vaginal insertion of any kind during pregnancy. These cases are not common and are usually temporary until the issue resolves. This recommendation may be made to reduce infection risk or if there's an increased risk of premature labor.

The postpartum sexual hiatus is well known. Remember, this time is a time of healing and rejuvenating. Six weeks is not a hard number either; some women feel ready for sex sooner, and some would rather wait longer. When you do feel ready for sex again in the postpartum, start with yourself. Everything has come back together differently after being expanded and reshaped.

Having a baby does not mean you don't have a tight vagina! I'd like to shout it from the rooftops. The whole idea that your vagina is no longer suitable for a man to feel good in is ludicrous. The pressure to have a tight vagina is insane, and I'm just not here for it. Have a strong pelvic floor to support your posture, your health, your bladder and bowel control but don't work to strengthen your pelvic floor because you think it makes you worthy of having sex with him. Your partner is blessed to get to see your naked body. They are fortunate to get to be inside you, and if he would like to insist that your vagina be tighter, then I recommend you insist his penis be bigger.

You are worthy, sexy and stunning. Appreciate the bodies you get to explore, including your own, and expect nothing less than extreme gratitude for the gift of getting to be inside you.

Chapter Three
Not Part of the Plan

While making the baby is super fun, sometimes it wasn't exactly part of the plan. One summer I locked my keys in my car eight times. If that was not an indicator that learning from my mistakes is not my best characteristic, then three unplanned pregnancies might tell you something. I've been there. Nothing throws a wrench in your plans for world domination quite like a positive pregnancy test.

When I was nineteen years old, I thought I had the flu—for two months—and obviously missed my period because I was stressed, right? When falling asleep in class became a regular thing, my professor pulled me aside and asked if I was struggling with pregnancy.

"What? Pregnant? Me?" Long, thinking pause. "Oh, shit."

I hear you. I know that overwhelming stress. During my third unplanned pregnancy, I contemplated suicide. Go ahead, throw a fit, be really frustrated, pissed off, guilty, embarrassed, worried, stressed, overwhelmed and downright terrified. Cry it out.

Okay, now it's big girl shoes time. Hair up, belly out. Let's do this.

First you make that big choice: keep it or don't. For some women, there's not a choice to make; they already know. This is not a chapter about pregnancy termination. I have been put on this earth to care for people and babies and to pet all the dogs. Judging your choices is not my calling. Just be ready to face the consequences, no matter the choice. Be brave and charge ahead, knowing you can face this big thing, even if you're going it alone.

During your pregnancy, your baby needs ten blissful minutes a day. Ten minutes of good, happy hormones passing through your placenta and building your baby's hormone receptors. Give yourself and your baby ten minutes a day. Most of the time, you'll build on these ten minutes. Ten minutes of a pleasant walk turns into thirty. Ten minutes of reading a book by your favorite author (it's me, we know) turns into an hour. Find bubbles of joy in this journey you're carrying around with you.

When a pregnancy is unplanned, every mildly annoying pregnancy symptom seems a lot worse. A little low back pain is, "My back hurts. I feel like a cow. I have enough gas, I'm about to put hazmat stickers on my ass. I'm broke and my back hurts!"

Let's try this again:

"Mama, how ya doing?" your midwife asks.

"I've been having some back pain, but I noticed if I stretch or roll on a massage ball, it feels better."

You had a problem; you tried something simple to make it manageable. No more wallowing. Be upset and then get up and do something about it.

This mental shift is sometimes hard to make. Putting a positive spin on things or having an I-got-this approach is not an easy thought pattern to create, but it's worth it, just for the pleasure of living.

Take it from someone who's been there—three freaking times, people—nothing will motivate you more than having to show up for another human. I recently rode a bicycle thirty-eight miles in five hours, not because I'm a well-trained cyclist who does this recreationally. No, in fact, prior to this trek, I had not spent more than an hour on a stationary bike in my tv room while I watched The Bachelor. But, because my son thought it would be fun, I repeat, I pedaled thirty-eight miles, hills and all, and was laid up and limping for three days . . . because my son wanted to . . . for funsies. When I tell you our kids will bring us to do things we never thought we'd do,

I am indisputably serious. I am my-right-knee-will-never-forgive-me serious.

This child is a call to action. It's time to rise. Get your life together, go make your money; you have a life to support. Get healthy, get a job, get a good partner, move to a better neighborhood, get a car that doesn't require three tries and a prayer to start, go, fight, win! You will never love anything the same way. Even in your struggles, you are enough for this baby. The hard parts are there for a reason; just keep walking forward, one step at a time. Motherhood is the toughest hood that ever existed, and you are the baddest mofo on the block.

Chapter Four
The Midwives

Once you are pregnant, or maybe before if you're proactive, you will want to choose a care provider. I'm keeping it basic but please ask questions or do more research on this as it sparks your interest.

Most people recognize the American standard of obstetrician. These are doctors who specialize in maternity care, labor and birth. Family practice doctors and doctors of osteopathic medicine can also catch babies and manage pregnancy complications if they have received adequate training to do so.

Midwives come in different types, mostly having to do with the education route the individual chose.

Certified Nurse Midwives (CNM), or nurse midwife for short, start with nursing school and then attend advanced training to learn maternity care, labor and birth as a specialty. Nurse midwives sometimes work with an obstetrician or in a solo practice, can prescribe medications and are nationally recognized. Some CNMs catch babies in hospitals, others work in birth centers and some attend home births.

Certified Professional Midwives (CPM) are more often considered "traditional" midwives. They meet the requirements of the North American Registry of Midwives (NARM) in order to take their national exam and be granted certification. As of this writing, there are two ways to meet the NARM requirements; one is by attending a midwifery school. Some of these schools are accredited by the Midwifery Education Accreditation Council (MEAC). The other option is the Portfolio Evaluation Process which means the midwife meets certain apprenticeship and education requirements in order to sit for the exam. Even though NARM is a national organization, CPMs are not recognized in every state. Currently, seven states have made traditional midwifery illegal: Kentucky, Alabama, Illinois, Iowa, Nebraska, North Carolina and South Dakota. In the other forty-three states, CPMs are regulated in a variety of ways or are alegal (neither illegal or regulated under any law).

Licensed Midwives (LM) take the NARM exam and become a CPM, then meet the requirements of their state to be granted a license in that state. How LMs are regulated and what they are permitted to do varies from state to state. There used to be more LMs and CPMs working in hospitals or clinics, but as the obstetric care model took over, these traditional midwifery care models were pushed out. Now LMs and CPMs attend births at birth centers or in homes.

For more in-depth history of maternity care, midwives, obstetricians and birth, I enjoyed the book Lying In: A History of Childbirth in America by Richard Wertz, but other books go deep into this topic as well.

A long time ago, midwives were the only ones going to births around the world. Pregnancy and birth were a woman's arena, and men were mostly not allowed in. Then a man recognized the opportunity to monetize birth. Don't get me wrong; before this dude, midwives were being paid with goods or money, but they were charging a fraction of what it later became.

A big, societal push came about that said pain, suffering and trials are bad! Never hurt! Oh no! Not the pain of childbirth! A woman should never suffer such pain!

But hold up. This was also when women were told, "Lay on your back, don't move, PUSH! Not fast enough! Here, I'll do it!" A rather painful way to birth!

Doctors took an "I can deliver this baby better than the mother can" approach. Experimental drugs, procedures and many, many deaths followed. Regulations came down on midwives, keeping them from doing their jobs and decreasing their numbers, not to mention the whole witch-hunt stigma that continued long after the Salem Witch Trials. Many midwives were murdered if a baby was born with a problem. People claimed the midwife was a witch and caused the defect.

While the exam required to become a certified professional midwife is administered by a national organization, every state in the U.S. is different with regard to how CPMs can practice. Some states are midwife-friendly and have thus increased the number of midwives practicing there. Other states make it illegal, don't regulate at all or make it difficult to practice midwifery in a sustainable way; therefore, these states have fewer midwives and fewer options for healthy moms.

No matter what type of care you start with, be aware that sometimes a person will begin their pregnancy care with a midwife, planning a home birth, but as the pregnancy progresses, conditions might arise that make it safer to birth in a hospital. This is part of the risk assessment that midwives do with their clients throughout care. No midwife should ever guarantee an out-of-hospital birth; they can only promise to be the guardian of safe birth and autonomy.

Doulas (pronounced doo-la) are not midwives, but they are part of the picture of birth and are becoming more common, especially as insurance starts to cover their services. Doulas are not medically trained. I adore a good doula and appreciate when a family has decided to hire one for their birth. However, certification is not required to be a doula. They are not regulated and neither is their training. There are organizations that provide training and certification if an individual should seek it, but it is not required under any law.

I've watched people scammed by a person who claimed to be a doula, took their money and then didn't show up to their birth, just straight ghosted them. A good doula has a contract explaining what she/he offers and charges and other policies like what happens if they miss your birth. Doulas provide emotional, mental and physical support during pregnancy, labor and postpartum. Some doulas take pictures, offer massage, provide warm compresses, counter pressure, aroma therapy, communicate with hospital staff as an advocate for you and give your partner breaks. That's just during labor. There are postpartum doulas who help you get more sleep, rest, nourishment and stay sane while adjusting to your new baby. Labor can be a marathon; doulas are your cheering squad, running alongside you, holding out water cups. (I recently learned that sometimes marathon runners poop themselves during the race, and this makes my comparison of labor to marathons even more accurate!) I encourage everyone to consider interviewing doulas and seeing if anyone fits. It's like hiring a friend who will encourage you to pee, poop and push.

I'll close this chapter with this thought. Beyond the education and paperwork that makes us midwives, I also clearly understand that the place I take in your pregnancy, labor and birth story is sacred. For many families I have stood in the doorway between life and death, raised a flat hand in the face of death and said, "not ta-day."

I am currently blessed to attend mostly home births. This means families don't just open their homes to me, they expose their bodies, their deepest fears, their families and their flaws. They invite me into their most vulnerable state and that makes me overwhelmingly grateful. I love to laugh and joke, but this part I take very seriously. It's an honor to be trusted with your baby, your wife, your partner and your life. Any behavior that reflects something different, I'm just not here for.

Chapter Five

The First Trimester

I could use the word symptom, as in pregnancy symptoms, but the definition of symptom is in relationship to disease. Pregnancy is not a disease; it's a life stage, a normal process. Instead of symptoms, these are fun little pregnancy shenanigans, treats, snippets or, for those of you down-to-earth gals, pregnancy fuckery.

Indications you might be pregnant or first trimester treats: nausea, restlessness, cramping, bloating, vomiting, frequent urination, change in body odor, oily skin, increase in acne, sore breasts, fatigue, spotty vaginal bleeding, increased smell sensitivity, increased flexibility, brain fog, heartburn, being gassy, changes in bowel movements, metallic taste and stuffy nose. Did I make pregnancy sound super fun? These are common and normal, but that doesn't make them any less annoying sometimes.

Of course, you can and should always talk to your midwife or care provider about how you're feeling physically and emotionally. Some treats can be reduced by increasing certain vitamins, changes in lifestyle or changes in hygiene products. Most women experience two or three treats from this list or something totally new—that's still normal. Some women don't experience any of these little gifts, and the unfortunate few go through a lot of these or extremes of these. Most first trimester goodies resolve or become more manageable as pregnancy goes on.

There's no need to sugar coat it: feeling dragged down in the first trimester by the pregnancy you were so excited about or completely unprepared for can suck. I know what you're thinking. "What are you talking about, Dev? I've been wanting to vomit in parking lots because of the smell of a fast-food restaurant! Who doesn't want to feel bloated and exhausted all day long?"

If any of your initial pregnancy signs suddenly stop or something just feels off to you, contact your midwife.

I like to see the first trimester as every woman's opportunity to set boundaries and offer herself grace. You can say no. Read that again: you can say no. Say it out loud. "I can say no."

No, I'm not going to the grocery store again, this week—hello delivery app. No, you can't use that shampoo anymore, husband of mine. Deal with it.

You can also try yes for balance. Yes, I will take my third nap today. Yes, I will eat another molasses cookie, because it's the only thing that sounds good right now. Yes, I am pregnant. Say it with me. "My body is ah-mazing. My body was designed perfectly. I know what my body needs. I'm allowed to be happy that I'm pregnant and cranky that I don't physically feel awesome. Being cranky doesn't make me a bad mom or unworthy of this pregnancy. I am worthy, I am enough, I am full of love."

While you are assessing and establishing boundaries on how other people treat you, have you noticed how you treat yourself? Do you give yourself time off? Take yourself out to do some of your favorite things? Do you offer yourself grace for this huge change in your body and your life? Do you do things that are healthy for you? Have you taken yourself to the dentist? Massage therapist? Hair stylist? Do you have an elaborate skin care routine that has gone by the wayside since you started having kids? My love, it's time. You've been waiting for you to love you, and you've been waiting to come home to yourself. (You've been waiting to see how many times I can use the word you in a single sentence, you, you, you, you.)

You are no stranger to transitioning. You transitioned as you grew up, as your body developed, as your family changed, as your

31

desires shifted, as you decided what you wanted to be when you grew up and then changed your mind, as you fell in love with a human and as you experienced heartbreak. You have transitioned many times, but when we are young and sometimes even when we are grown, we aren't always given direction on how to manage those transitions. Becoming pregnant is a transitional period. You are no longer the past you. No matter how this pregnancy turns out, when it first comes, it changes you. It's okay to mourn; there is loss of the former you, a former life, a former thought pattern. Mourning a change does not mean you are not grateful or ready for it. There is a piece of you that felt safe and content in that former state, and that piece feels skeptical of the unknown, because it wants to protect you. Hug that piece of yourself, tell her it's okay, you got this. It's safe to be pregnant; it's safe to be someone new. Growth is safe, and growth is magical.

I want to relay an important message. Duality is normal. Duality is safe, perfect, loving, genuine and wonderful. You can be grateful for what you have and still want more. You can be mad that you feel crappy and still love your baby, your body and the fact that you're pregnant. You do not have to feel guilty for any negative feelings that come up about being pregnant. Sometimes it sucks, sometimes it freakin' rocks. Wanting to be alone does not make you a bad partner or mother or friend. Neither does wanting attention, love, respect or deep connection. You can be both sad and grateful at the same time. You can be disappointed and strong and ready at the same time. We are complex, badass, loving, inspiring, strong, capable women. In the words of Alanis Morisette, "I'm free but I'm focused, I'm green, but I'm wise, I'm hard but I'm friendly, baabay, I'm sad but I'm laughing, I'm brave but I'm chicken sh**. . ."

When you start interviewing for the maternity care provider of your dreams, you will find that not all care providers do consults or interviews. If you want to meet them, you have to schedule and pay for an appointment with them. Many midwives I know offer consultations—sometimes free consults—but not all of them, so call or message and ask.

The initiation of care does not necessarily have to be in the first trimester, this just happens to be where I decided to talk about it. There are some benefits to initiating care early in your pregnancy but don't over stress if time got away from you or if you didn't realize you were pregnant until later. From the beginning, there is an onslaught of decisions to make, and yes, they are your decisions. Just because it's routine care does not mean it's required or necessary.

To determine how far along you are, a care provider might request a dating ultrasound. These can be helpful if you have irregular periods, or don't know the date of conception, because you and your man just get down whenever there is a slight breeze (you go, girl). Knowing how far along you are helps your care provider know when you and your baby are hitting certain benchmarks for growth and that you are not delivering prematurely. Some practitioners refer for a dating ultrasound routinely, even if you know your menstrual cycle and/or conception date. This referral comes out of the CYA (cover your ass) mentality.

The dating ultrasound can also confirm an intrauterine pregnancy with a live baby, ruling out ectopic pregnancy, molar pregnancy, chemical pregnancy or other complications that mimic pregnancy signs. These complications are not common, but if left unchecked, they can cause serious problems. If there is any alarm or concern, seek immediate care. Some people prefer to avoid medical intervention as much as possible and that means passing on what is not immediately necessary. Ultrasound is not completely without risk, as ultrasounds use sound waves that heat and affect cells. This is why many professionals, the FDA and the WHO recommend against serial ultrasounds and caution against prolonged ultrasounds. There are alternative ways to estimate a due date, including assessing your menstrual cycle and feeling for your fundal height, which is the length from pubic bone to the top of your uterus. Weighing the risks and the benefits is very personal and requires your determination.

Typically when you begin care, your provider wants to order blood work. Initial lab testing gives your care provider a look into your overall health and helps them create a plan for you based on the results. We'll start with the pregnancy panel, this includes blood type, rh factor, antibody screen, complete blood count, testing for syphilis, hepatitis B, Rubella and HIV. A urine sample testing for UTI, gonorrhea and chlamydia is also standard. In addition to this, many care providers are now also adding thyroid tests, vitamin B12, vitamin D and ferritin, as well.

That was a lot of me listing off diseases and letters so let's break it down real quick. An obstetric panel is routine because all the diseases being tested for could cause negative outcomes, but if addressed early, that risk can be reduced. Blood typing is important because of the slight chance of ABO incompatibility, which is when an A, B, O or AB blood type mixes with a different type and causes an immune response. Think of it like an allergic reaction to a blood type. This is rare but serious. Blood typing also checks for the possibility of Rh isoimmunization, which only happens if the mother is Rh negative and the baby is Rh positive and their blood mixes. It's also valuable to have your blood type in the chart just in case you need a blood transfusion—not a common occurrence.

A complete blood count (CBC) is such a cool thing, in my opinion. This is an assessment of the basic makeup of your blood, what portion of your blood is white blood cells and red blood cells, and how many hundreds of thousands of platelets you have per cubic millimeter. The other numbers in a CBC give information about the size, shape, type and oxygen content of those cells. Hemoglobin and hematocrit stand out to most practitioners when reading a CBC. Simply put, hemoglobin is the amount of oxygen in red blood cells while hematocrit is what percentage of your blood is red blood cells. These numbers can tell a care provider whether or not you are anemic, what stage of an infection you are in (if you have one), whether or not you are iron deficient, B12 deficient or neither, and wave other pink/red flags that indicate further examination. The CBC is so cool because it tells a story. It can change throughout your day, your cycle, your pregnancy, with changes in your diet, your hydration level, your stress level, even based on where you live. If I have clients who can't afford the plethora of testing done in early pregnancy, I typically encourage at least a CBC; it's usually inexpensive, even without insurance, and gives valuable information to move forward.

It's helpful if you over-share. Knowing how you're feeling and all the things your body is experiencing helps your provider make an informed decision on what labs to request. Yes, she does want to know that your boobs are sore, and one is bigger than the other. Yes, she does want to know that your vagina smells different, you have back acne, and you're angry about everything. You are fascinating, exciting and unique—share away! Your health and overall body function is bigger than your pregnancy, but many women don't make a regular health visit if they aren't pregnant, which makes prenatal visits an opportunity to check in on you and maybe catch something that could affect you outside of pregnancy.

Allow me to give you a little background on ferritin, which just sounds like a sophisticated name for a cat. Serum ferritin was discovered in the 1930s. A test to quantify ferritin came about in the 70s. The value of ferritin testing came into widespread discussion in obstetrics around 2010, as far as I can tell. Today, research suggests that assessing ferritin throughout pregnancy should be the industry standard. Ferritin is a protein that stores iron which means the ferritin number on your lab results equates to the amount of iron you have stored up in your body just waiting to be moved to a usable form of iron. Your body needs this to maintain healthy iron levels as your blood volume and body expand, as your placenta places a greater demand on your body to get through labor and to recover from birth. Looking at ferritin levels is like getting a peek into the future of how you might maintain energy during labor, bleed immediately after the birth and recover after birthing. When we look into the crystal ball of lab results, a low ferritin level can also be an indicator that anemia will occur later in pregnancy.

Have you peed in a cup lately? What? You haven't been training for the American Cup Urination Event? Well, strap in, Buttercup, 'cause you're about to start practice. Some providers check your urine at every visit, so make it fun. Put the cup on the floor, strip naked and buy yourself ice cream if you make it in the cup! (I'm kidding, please don't do that at my office.)

Most providers at least get a urine sample from you at the start of care and then maybe not again unless a symptom or concern arises. The first visit collection is usually for testing for gonorrhea, chlamydia, a urinary tract infection (UTI) and possibly a pregnancy confirmation test. Gonorrhea and chlamydia can cause pre-term labor, newborn infection or other complications, so the sooner either one is identified and treated, the better. Your care provider doesn't know you; they aren't trying to offend you or your partner by taking these tests. They are simply covering their bases, and they'd rather test and get a negative than not test when a person is positive.

Many women don't experience symptoms of a UTI while pregnant, although women are more susceptible to them while pregnant, because hormones give the urethra permission to be lazy, and the urethra is like a working mom with two kids in soccer and one in gymnastics. She's been waiting for that permission to relax. This chillin' can cause bacteria to build up in certain areas. This is one reason it's pertinent to drink plenty of water and urinate when you have the urge. UTIs often go unnoticed in pregnancy, because the main symptom is frequent urination, which you have anyway, because your baby is using your bladder as a pillow or a bean bag chair—shout out to the breech babes!

At this point, I'm talking a lot about stuff that happens in the bathroom. Girl, just move in there; get some pillows and orange juice in a champagne flute and live in your bathroom. Happy baby growing, be blessed.

You can decline any and all of these tests as much or as little as you want, for whatever reason you want. It's not your care providers job to make you do anything. They are there to provide care (duh) and give you options. You can request a print-out of results and track your own numbers over time. This is valuable for getting a picture of what is normal for you. If you want extra tests, you can request that as well. Go ahead, be powerful and in charge of your health. Watch you work!

Chapter Six
Trauma and Pregnancy

This chapter begins with a trigger warning for sexual abuse and partner violence. If these things are triggering for you, then please skip this chapter. You don't have to know the details; just know I've been there, and I'm here with you. If this is possibly triggering for you, stop reading here.

I endured sexual, emotional and physical abuse for almost ten years at the hands of people who were deeply influential and connected to me. However, I do not believe that my suffering was redemptive. I don't believe that I was being punished for something. I do not believe that because I have suffered, I'm now worthy of a better life nor that I was deserving of the suffering. I was born worthy of a good, abundant, happy life. I am redeemed through my actions of growth and better choices. This happened to me, and it doesn't mean anything about me. I am not less than, or dirty, or in any way living in shame because of what happened to me. Shame is not for me. You too were born worthy. We are worthy of moving on and moving up.

My personal example of a trauma response during pregnancy looks like this: During my third pregnancy, from about thirty weeks on, my baby sat low in my pelvis and occasionally moved against a spot deep inside me that sent me into a spiral of crying and panic. This spot was clearly where I held previous trauma. Maybe it was the actual spot pressed during one of the rapes, maybe it was emotionally holding on to the feeling of touch violations, maybe it was connected to the nerves stimulated by fear in the whoosie-whats-it part of my brain! Who knows. All I know is when I felt pressure there, my brain immediately recognized it as a danger and set off alarms.

My subconscious screamed, Run! Don't let that happen! Panic! It's happening again! That hurts us!

So you know what I did? I embraced it. Every time my baby hit that spot, I felt the panic bubble up, and I cried. I let it out, and I repeated out loud, "You're safe. Your baby is safe. This feeling is safe."

I moved all my mental energy to that sensation and imagined my baby inside of me, rubbing his adorable head against my muscles like it felt good for him. I hugged my belly and breathed into the sensation. I also used EFT (Emotional Freedom Technique, a tapping method) throughout that pregnancy under the guidance of a specialist. This was after three years of therapy and eye movement desensitization and reprocessing (EMDR) to cope with and manage my PTSD episodes pre-pregnancy. It has taken a lot of work to get to a place where I can recognize trauma responses and change my reaction. It's an everyday kind of work.

For me, home birth was a birth with choices. For me, both my home births made me feel capable and empowered. They brought me back to being the owner of my body. Through a positive experience with birth, my vagina and the abilities of my body, I was able to reclaim the body that was taken from me as a teenager.

Where you choose to birth might be influenced by your trauma. You might feel safest in the hospital where you have every tool available to you. A birth center might feel cozy and safe to you, in the trusted hands of a care provider who knows what you need. The comfort of your home can also feel good. This is a personal decision that can change throughout your pregnancy as things develop.

In my experience, denying trauma, pushing it away and "soldiering on" doesn't serve us in the long term and especially not in birth. Birth has a way of reaching inside us and pulling it out. Talk about your fears, your traumas, your hesitations and your insecurities. Drag them out by their ankles and face them! This doesn't mean you should replay the traumatic experience in your mind over and over again. I'm suggesting you take a long hard look at how the trauma is affecting you. How has it influenced your choices? Are you reacting to situations from your trauma?

Acknowledging how your trauma is affecting your decisions, reactions, thoughts and behavior is an important step towards improvement and healing. Talk to the right people, the specialists, the holistic healers, the whole body, mind, spirit searchers and the optimists. Create a safe space for you to address the traumatic experiences you've faced. Prepare for not everyone to be available to help you through it, and I don't just mean time in their schedule but energetically available. Some people aren't ready to honor your journey; they have to deal with their own trauma, and that's okay.

Your mental health is important during every part of your pregnancy. Depression is not just for the postpartum. Prenatal depression is a real thing, so is prenatal anxiety. There are nutritional steps you can take to feed your body the nutrients that help it make more favorable brain chemistry for fighting depression. Talk therapy is also great but not your only option. Tapping, acupuncture, journaling, Reiki, massage, EMDR, yoga, stretching, meditation, podcasts, books and time outside in the sunshine are all healthy therapy options that are safe in pregnancy when done/taught by someone trained in pregnancy safe techniques.

Your midwife should be informed of and sensitive to your history. This helps your care provider know how best to respect you during your pregnancy, labor and birth. It also helps give you full control. Sometimes just getting this out in the open is preventative. Like I said, birth brings it all out anyway, so get real with yourself and your team.

There are a lot of different types of trauma and ways to be traumatized. A previous birth experience could have been difficult or unexpected. A previous pregnancy loss or a friend or family member's experience can linger in your mind (another reason it's important to be selective about who you share your story with. Those with expertise and practice guarding their energy are best suited to be the most helpful and not take on your trauma themselves).

Moving can cause trauma; a pandemic, a divorce, a death, or any life changing event can stir up emotions and come back up later. There's nothing wrong with these things; they are part of our growth and part of our development. They're healthy and how we build a life. These experiences do not get to own you. They don't get to take away the joy you are meant to experience.

We are meant to give ourselves grace, set boundaries and recognize when we need more time to adjust to the change(s). Hug the parts of you that want to keep you safe using fear and hiding. Tell them it's okay to move forward. What's on the other side is everything beautiful that belongs to you. You are safe, you are not alone, and you are worthy of deep healing.

Chapter Seven

What Are You Putting in Your Mouth?

Pregnancy is an indescribable journey that is unique to each person involved. So much of pregnancy, labor, birth and postpartum can feel out of our control, but that dismissive thinking is not for you. Our daily habits are the steppingstones up or down the mountain of good health. There is no one-size-fits-all exercise routine and nutrition plan. Often, the only way to learn your ideal good health habits is by trial and error. Hopefully this chapter will serve as a jumping off point or a nudge in the right direction.

Let's start from the beginning. No, not the "yea, you're pregnant" part—before that. You've decided to get pregnant (unless you didn't, in which case, start now anyway). Take this opportunity to up-level your life, starting with your nutrition. A good prenatal vitamin is great, but it's not the end-all, be-all.

Your prenatal care should have forms of vitamins that are easy for your body to digest, such as methylated B12 or methylcobalamin versus unmethylated B12 or cyanocobalamin which is harder for your body to break down. Avoid artificial sweeteners as much as possible. In the first trimester, you get a pass if you can only stomach the gummy vitamins; they're better than nothing. Here's why prenatal vitamins are not enough—they were designed to replace just what your baby is skimming off the top from your body. The flaw is that this is the bare minimum for the survival of a baby. While a vitamin specific to pregnancy has been a great moneymaker for manufactures,

41

it doesn't begin to cover the nutrient demands of your life that is filled with other kids, a job, a partner, environmental pollution and other factors that have left you depleted before you even got pregnant. You deserve more than survival, my love. You can strive for optimal. It's important to give your body AND your baby an abundance of nutrients, store up for the work of labor, birth and postpartum and come back from the deficiencies of your past.

Most prenatal vitamins don't contain healthy fats which your baby and your placenta love! A good fish oil, flax seed oil or avocado oil supplement is also important. The dose may vary per individual, but it's often higher than you think, depending on your dietary intake and needs. If your diet is rich in these fats, then you can go lower in a supplemental dose, but it's recommended to cut back on fish consumption to reduce mercury intake during pregnancy.

Vitamin C is great for your infection fighting abilities and potentially for reducing GBS colonization (more on that later).

Probiotics are important for good gut health, which is an essential part of nutrient absorption, herbal treatment effectiveness, immune system function and regulation of bacteria growth.

All supplements are not created equal. If it's important to you, then you should research a company that strikes your interest. Do the ethics of the company sit well with you? Some companies source their products or packaging differently, so if you're searching for something that is, for example, American-made or plant-based, some research might be required.

It's true what they say: Some supplements are just expensive pee. You want supplements that your body can actually absorb and use without all the extra fluff, dyes and artificial sweeteners. Learn how to read labels. I recommend that my clients check the label to make sure the B12 and folate in a supplement is a methylated form, like I mentioned earlier. Without doing a major deep dive I'll briefly explain.

Research suggests that half of the US population has an MTHFR mutation. MTHFR (I lovingly refer to this as the Motha Fuckr) is an enzyme. When mutated, it inhibits the way your body breaks down homocysteine (an amino acid). This means it can build up in your system and become toxic, which causes a variety of conditions. MTHFR mutations have been linked to cardiovascular disease, thromboembolism, depression, anxiety, bipolar disorder, schizophrenia, colon cancer, acute leukemia, chronic pain, chronic fatigue, migraines, recurrent miscarriages and neural tube defects in unborn babies. More research is needed, and there are variants that require even more research.

Here's what we know: These problems suck—and this part is important—they could potentially be resolved or worsened because of what you eat! Methylated B12 methylcobalamin and methylfolate are already broken down, which means if someone happened to have an MTHFR mutation, this is a usable B12 source for them versus one that they can't break down. If a person does not have an MTHFR mutation and still takes a methylated form of B12, they don't get superpowers, they get their B12. I highly recommend reviewing MTHFR with your provider. Changing how you eat could change your life.

Prenatal vitamins usually have something like 500-2000 International Units (IUs) of vitamin D, but most people in North America are deficient, and this dose isn't enough to make up for that. You may be among the people who need significantly more D (the vitamin and the other thing). For optimal pregnancy health, 10,000 IUs is more appropriate.

Some women need to take an iron supplement, but most prenatal vitamins do not contain iron because of the risk of toxicity. After your initial lab work, your care provider will tell you if you need to supplement iron. If you opt out of lab work, then your risk factors combined with your symptoms will help determine if you should supplement iron. Like the others, not all iron supplements are created equal; some are constipating. Constipation is not a sign that you are taking too much, but it is a sign that you may need a different supplement or a different environment to take it in.

For example, you may need to add a probiotic to your supplement regimen to give yourself the best gut flora for breaking down iron.

You also want to check your other supplements; calcium and iron compete for absorption, so don't take them together. Vitamin C helps with iron absorption so take those together. Your body digests best when you are at rest and not stressed, so take your iron when you're chill (that's right I said you have to chill at some point).

Unfortunately, we can't have custom-made prenatal vitamins (yet), so you will probably have to mix and match different supplements to get everything your unique, wonderful, gorgeous body needs. If this means you don't take a prenatal at all, that's okay too. Besides, and I can't stress this enough, your real nutrients come from what you eat, not that row of pills you're poppin'. Find your sweet spot. Some people function better on gluten free, some people thrive as a meat eater, and some people feel the best as a vegetarian. We are all so beautifully and uniquely made, honor your individuality by feeding your body what it needs.

That's the basics. Your care provider may recommend other supplements as things come up such as magnesium, iron, calcium and a variety of herbs/teas.

While you're adding supplements and healthy foods, you may also need to be taking away. Let's use common sense here. You know that glazed pastry is not good for you. You know going through the fast-food line, again, is not the healthiest choice. Your four pump, quad shot with caramel drizzle is not good for you! Your body is on loan to you. When you're done, you have to give it back, and it will only go as long as it can. If you give your body love, care, honor and respect, it will love you back.

Remember the food industry is a trickster. They can write "natural" on a box, if at one point, some ingredient somewhere was natural. Sometimes we believe that sitting in front of the T.V. binge eating ice cream is self-care or self-love. Let me ask you this. If your child, who you love unconditionally, was plowing through a gallon of chocolate-chip-cookie-dough, would you want that for them? Or would you rather see them enjoy a fresh salad and get to bed on time? We want our children to live long, healthy lives. Why don't we want that for ourselves? I mean really want it, enough to be disciplined for it. Eating well is true love.

Our emotions are governed by hormones. Our body's ability to produce happy hormones is greatly impacted by what we eat. This fact is unpopular because it puts the ball back in your court. You can blame genetics, global warming, politics, religion, your circumstances and the universe all you want Sugar, nothing changes the fact that considering pasta your main food group can cause depression, anxiety and generally feeling unhappy. Hormones control us; they make us attracted to our mate or some random person at the grocery store who looks good in "dem jeans" today. Cortisol makes us stressed and amped up; oxytocin makes us whimsical and in love. Estrogen makes us willing to serve; progesterone says, "Nah, the kids are fine, go get a massage." Of course, we also have some testosterone that walks around with too much confidence and says, "Hey, nice truck."

I feel an animated film featuring Cortisol, Oxytocin, Estrogen, Progesterone and Testosterone coming on. Hormones are substances within your body; these substances need building blocks to be made—building blocks that come from food. When moms tell me they are prone to postpartum depression, the first place I look is their diet. Thyroid, pancreas, mood swings, feeling overwhelmed, hyper-fixated, worrying all the time—the issues with these things circle back to hormone imbalances that can quite often (not every single time) be helped or fixed with a change in food choices. I won't completely write off environmental factors, but we also have at least some control over our environment. In fact, probably more control than you think you have.

Check your excuses and take ownership of your food intake. I'm reminded of the quote by Thomas Edison, "Opportunity is missed by most people because it comes dressed in overalls and looks like work" (even though his ethics were questionable).

Pick protein-rich foods, vegetables and healthy fats first and move your body in ways that feel good. I hope that good nutrition and healthy exercise is something you repeatedly revisit throughout your life.

Some women become anemic during their pregnancy because two things are at play: (1) their body is using iron and other minerals to support their placenta, growing uterus, stretching tissues and baby or babies, and (2) their blood is becoming hemodiluted. I've heard it said that your blood volume will double during pregnancy—not quite. Your body is, in fact, adding half of the liquid portion of your blood. Put simply, your blood will be watered down. This means that a sample of blood taken at twenty-eight weeks into your pregnancy will have fewer cells in it than a sample taken at eight weeks. So, when you say you feel water-logged and bloated, you're a mermaid. Go with it.

Because of hemodilution, some decrease in lab values is normal, but there are still lower limits. You can counteract these blood level drops by increasing your nourishing foods. Dark, leafy greens are a recommended staple of most midwives along with red meat (unless meat is not your jam, that's cool. I refer back to dark, leafy greens), beets, sweet potatoes, quinoa and broccoli. There is some iron in dark chocolate (you're welcome).

Not only will your pregnancy soak up iron and dilute your blood, but that whole calcium-leeching thing you may have heard about is true. Your teeth may change, your eyesight, hair, skin pigment, hormones, digestion, bowel movements, mood, your body odor, fingernails, and yes, your sex drive are affected by nutrients and a lack thereof.

Drink water, drink water, drink water. Hey, drink more water! Being well hydrated prevents so much discomfort and keeps your body flowing, literally. Drinking water prevents Braxton-Hicks contractions, dry skin, dry mouth, dry nasal passages, dizziness, confusion, bags under your eyes, varicose veins, urinary tract infections, vaginal dryness, headache, constipation, thirst (duh), fatigue, overheating, low amniotic fluid and irritability. Wow, right? Drink water.

Since you are preparing for the marathon that is birth, you must train like an athlete, and that means consuming electrolytes. Have a seat while I take you back to ninth grade science class. Your body, every second of every day, seeks homeostasis. Homeo-what, you might ask. It is science-speak for perfect balance. If your body was not seeking balance, it would just let you keep bleeding when you get a paper cut or not slow your heart down after you've been startled. Our bodies keep us alive by constantly striving for homeostasis.

The balance of the fluids within our bodies is essential to the functioning of cells. Electrolytes are minerals that, when in water, become electrically charged ions. Electrolyte liquid is structured to balance the fluid that cross the cell membrane and fluid that is around cells. Some examples of electrolytes include sodium, chloride, bicarbonate, calcium, phosphate and magnesium. These should sound familiar if you've ever read a food label. It's possible to overconsume or under consume these nutrients. They are necessary, and you don't have to drink highly commercialized sports drinks to get adequate amounts. These minerals exist in produce, nuts, cheese, milk, pickled foods and good quality non-iodized salt. Electrolytes affect respiratory rate, heart function, kidney function, blood pressure, cancer development and cellular function in various ways.

To summarize, get off to a good start by taking your vitamins, staying hydrated and eating your vegetables. If you're already pregnant, it's never too late to show your body some love.

Chapter Eight

Boobs, Butts and Vaginas

Have I said it enough times? Every woman is unique, and every pregnancy is different, which means any of the following might occur and it might not. Just because I talk about them here does not mean that if this stuff doesn't happen to you, there's something wrong. It just means your body is doing things in its own way. It's all part of your beautiful uniqueness; embrace it.

Your boobs are nothing short of wild magic. They can also be weird. Throughout pregnancy, breasts can hurt, grow, shrink, leak, get hard, get soft (turns out it's not just for penises!), get lumpy and be extra sensitive. These changes can happen in any trimester. They can come and go, and they are perfectly normal. My best advice is to find a bra, bralette, or tank top that works the best for you and buy all of them or go bra-less all together; the judgy, general public can kick rocks.

If your boobs are leaking, don't panic. Most of the time, your body is preparing to feed your baby and just getting excited. The fluid is usually clear to a slight off-white tint. If the fluid is bloody, foul smelling, brown, green or thick like mayonnaise, reach out to your lactation consultant or care provider. I think it goes without saying that bleeding from the nipples is not normal, but I'm just making sure I let you know. If your breasts hurt too much to bear, avoid a hot compress during this time, because heat attracts fluid, and we don't need you more swollen. Sometimes breasts hurt due to an overproduction of progesterone. There are some gentle herbs to help balance you out a little. Consult your care provider for what is right for you.

Have we established that I love me some healthy boundaries? Sore breasts present yet another opportunity to set those boundaries. Set those boundaries like Oprah handing out books: "You get a boundary, and you get a boundary, and you get a boundary!"

If your boobs require a hands-off policy for your partner, so be it. Of course, address that with some understanding, because I can almost promise that your partner will forget, cop a feel and then feel bad when you cry out in pain. These are big changes for everyone; give each other grace and respect. Now, if your partner repeatedly crosses the boundary or refuses to abide by this new policy, it's time for a more serious conversation. It is your body, and you get to decide who touches it, even if they have been allowed to touch it before. You are allowed to set this boundary even if your breasts aren't sore; maybe you're just feeling less physically available.

Let's move on to your vagina—another body part that does not take into consideration that you have a life to live, a job, a family, a social life and a sex life. Throughout your pregnancy, your vagina might change smell, become swollen, produce extra fluid, produce less fluid, leak white milky stuff, leak clear stuff, leak sticky stuff, change color and be more sensitive. Doesn't this sound fun? If your vagina decides to be a little drier or not produce lubrication at the moment you would like it to, you may need to increase the amount of foreplay, oh darn (#sarcasm) or use a safe and trusted lubricant. During pregnancy, blood flow increases to your vagina, making it more sensitive and causing it to change color. You might even notice some spotting after sex because of this extra vascularity. Again, totally normal, and before you call your care provider in a panic because you saw blood, ask yourself, "Did I have sex lately?"

Regular stretching and position changes can help move the fluid around your body and reduce fluid pooling in any one place. This extra vaginal swelling can also cause some itching. It should not be excessive, and it should go away with increased movement/ stretching. Report itching, burning and other changes to your care provider, so you can work together to rule out infections.

The chemistry of your vagina changes in preparation to pass a baby through it. If you are having a planned C-section, sorry your vagina didn't get the memo. This does leave you more vulnerable to yeast and bacterial infections. Good hygiene goes a long way. Breathable cotton underwear, healthy food intake and a probiotic supplement can also be helpful to prevent these infections. Pay attention to what you put in your vagina. Gently inserting things into your vagina for pleasure is not a bad thing but make sure everything is properly cleaned.

It's not recommended to acquire a new sexual partner during pregnancy, but sometimes it just happens that way; I get it. Just be safe! Sexually transmitted infections during pregnancy are no joke. Some can be transferred to baby, and most of them increase the risk of premature birth. Don't mess around with this.

Should your vagina ever itch uncontrollably, produce a foul smell, produce a yellow, clear and/or runny, green, gray or cottage cheese-like substance, report this to your care provider and consider getting tested. Often testing for infections can be done with a swab of the vagina or a urine test. Some providers use a speculum for this swabbing, but as I mentioned before, your vagina may be extra sensitive. Unless a provider needs to visually inspect your cervix, a speculum is not necessary. Often the issue can be treated based on the description of symptoms alone, without the need for a physical exam. You are also capable of swabbing your own vagina. That's right, I said it. Just one more of the many tasks incredible you is capable of. Yea!

So hey, what's your butt hole been up to lately? But seriously, have you ever had hemorrhoids? No? Welcome to pregnancy. We fart when we don't want to, we pee when we laugh, and we get sore, swollen vessels on our rectum. Remember all that extra fluid I was talking about? This also effects what's called venous (vee-nus) return, which is the ability of your blood to flow back through your veins. This reduced flow can cause varicose veins on your legs, vagina and rectum.

Hemorrhoids may not appear until after rigorous pushing or pressure during birth or bowel movements. Have I given you enough to worry about? I hope it eases your mind to know these are normal, uncomfortable, but most often not excruciating. They are usually easily managed and do not indicate you will have any issue when not pregnant or that anything is wrong with your body. Making sure that your diet contains adequate fiber and hydration to reduce constipation, and avoid aggressive pushing when using the bathroom.

I just want to point out that I mentioned another thing that can be prevented or helped by eating healthy foods. Can I also get a dollar for every time I've talked about drinking enough water? It's important! If you happen to develop a hemorrhoid, witch hazel applied with a cotton ball, gauze or a slice of potato left on the hemorrhoid between trips to the bathroom can be helpful.

The point of this chapter is to remind you that many strange things can happen to your most personal areas, and while they are not life threatening, they can be uncomfortable and make your experience less than pleasant. That's valid. You're allowed to be annoyed and humbled by this pregnancy fuckery. There also might be times when you need to talk about what your body is doing because your care provider may have more questions. Trust your instincts; if something seems off, then say something. Your body is amazing. It changes in so many ways while pregnant, and you endure many glorious, odd happenings. As always, give yourself grace, have a sense of humor and be grateful that we live in a time of pantyliners, hemorrhoid creams and padded tank tops.

Chapter Nine

D is for Dollars

L et's talk money.

Whoa, Dev! It's a pregnancy empowerment book; why money?

Because someone has to pay for things! Let me go broad and say, if money is a stressful topic for you, address that. If you have some childhood wounds or religious imprint that tells you money is evil, bad, problematic, or scary, it's time to challenge that. Money is a resource; it works for you. There's more than enough to go around.

Who cares for you and where you birth are very personal decisions. It's my deepest wish for you that you can rise out of any financial situation and not be forced to make a decision that is not right for you solely because of money. Many midwives bill insurance, offer hardship discounts or negotiate payment plans. You don't know if you don't ask. Many CPMs and LMs don't work for a hospital or major conventional medical practice, so they don't have the luxury of being recognized by all insurance companies. Some insurances won't cover home birth or birth center births. Others don't recognize care providers other than a CNM or OB. Some insurance companies pay CPMs and LMs less than CNMs.

Discuss the financial side with your midwife because there are so many ways to make a payment plan work for everyone. Let's discuss some terms that might come up.

Global fee covers certain parts of the standard maternity schedule care, including such things as gathering your health history, a physical exam, gathering vitals on you and baby, visits every four weeks until twenty-eight weeks, every two weeks until thirty-six weeks and every week until birth, management of uncomplicated labor and birth, repair of a first or second degree tear if necessary, delivery of placenta and routine postpartum visits.

What a global fee does not cover (based on most insurances): confirmation of pregnancy, visits outside of the usual schedule, non-stress test ultrasound, biophysical profile, lab tests, early labor observation, repair of third or fourth degree tear, management of delayed postpartum hemorrhage, management of mastitis, management of infection and any newborn care.

Just because it's not included in the global fee doesn't mean it isn't covered by your insurance. This is just what is encompassed or left out of this term. When your midwife says, "This is my global fee," be aware that she can bill separately for anything outside of a global fee.

You can also ask any care provider what their global fee is, then ask your insurance how much a global maternity fee they cover, and you'll have an idea of what you can expect to pay for the bare minimum. If your care provider is in-network or has experience billing your particular insurance, they can probably tell you what your insurance will cover and what you will owe for the global. Also be aware, the global fee is billed at the end of your care—six weeks postpartum—because insurance companies won't look at a bill for something that hasn't been done yet. Which means your insurance might not pay out until a few months after your birth.

Cap fee is the absolute most a client will pay. No matter what your insurance pays, no matter what happens during your pregnancy or birth, if your midwife has a cap fee, she's saying that is the most she will charge you, period. The practice you choose to care for you while you are pregnant should provide you with a financial agreement which outlines what exceptions might exist that aren't covered by the cap fee. For example, some midwives don't include newborn care. Read the financial policies/agreement thoroughly for the fees that aren't covered under the cap fee. Ask how they are covered. By insurance? By you?

The disparities in insurance billing and pay-outs between hospital and home birth are huge. This means that out-of-hospital birth is generally cheaper for the client. Check your insurance coverage; traditional midwives might be in-network for you or work with a CNM who is. Check your out-of-network coverage and your maternity care coverage. If you don't have insurance, but you are currently shopping for it, look for a policy with out-of-network coverage AND maternity care coverage. You don't want to be limited by your insurance if you find the care provider you want, but they are out-of-network.

When you find yourself stressing about the money, make a list of things you are grateful for. Don't roll your eyes—it works! You'll feel better and more aware of what you have. You are resourceful. Get creative about how you can change your financial situation. Trust that you can achieve all that you want. Pray that the money will come and then do the work.

Chapter Ten

Second Trimester

Let's talk second trimester, from fourteen weeks to twenty-seven weeks and six days. Hopefully some of the first trimester shenanigans are easing up on you. This is the part of pregnancy where people joke about funny food cravings, and you start rocking cute clothes over your bump. Some moms have stated that this is also when strangers think they can randomly touch your belly as though it isn't still part of your body. This seems to be less common as people catch on to the inappropriateness of it.

You'll be glowing, you'll be eating again, you'll have gorgeous, full boobs and you will hold all the power to create a tiny universe. Or maybe you aren't feeling glow-y and creator-of-life vibes; that's okay! It's okay to be moody, horny and sweaty. It's also okay to know that your growing uterus and the increase in progesterone flowing through your system are causing your metabolism to slow down, making you feel extra bloated and gassy. Sexy, right?

Good nutrition in this stage of pregnancy not only helps reduce some of pregnancy discomforts but also sets the stage for a smoother third trimester and a more favorable birth. Side note on that: I use the word favorable and other words with positive association, because words like easy, fast and painless are misleading and can lead to shaming when it comes to labor and birth. First off, since when is anything that changes your life ever easy? It's not easy and it's not supposed to be. It can be beautiful, wonderful, life changing, magical, graceful, peaceful and not as painful as you thought it would be, but it's not easy. Fast births can be nice, but they also shouldn't be every woman's focus.

Major, life-changing events happening fast can spiral into feelings of inadequacy, lack of control and shock rather than joy and comfort. It's not a bad thing for labor to take its time; babies can ease into the outside world gently. Babies need the time to adjust just as much as new parents do. Painless and tolerable are different. You will not hear me preaching painless birth—even though I'm familiar with many practitioners who do—because there is no shame in feeling pain! I'll circle back to this topic in the labor and birth chapter. Summary: good nutrition = energy for mom, strong well-nourished muscles and the ability to get through anything.

Good nutrition is not a diet. You should get a lot of calories and eat high doses of those good-for-you foods. "Hello, kale!"

So you hate kale, but have you tried kale chips? That's cool; you don't have to choke down foods you hate, just enjoy exploring things you are open to. Fortunately, we live in the wonderful age of supplements (providing that you don't skimp on quality) to make up some of the difference between your food intake and optimal health.

I know some of my readers won't like that statement. They'd rather I tell everyone to get all their nutrients from a whole foods diet. For many of us, eating a well-rounded, plentiful, natural diet of foods that contain just the amount of the nutrients we need every day is just not a reasonable expectation. Supplements are a miraculous gift for the modern woman. But be critical of the supplements you consider, you're worthy of the best.

Because your body didn't come with a manual, it's on you to do the research. Be an informed patient and get a college degree in your health. I suggest keeping a journal or at least a file of your medical records. Keep copies of your lab results. Track your cycle and other changes your body makes. Using your in-depth knowledge of yourself, you can work together with the care provider of your choice to help you live your best life. Your provider can and should help keep you accountable, give you guidance, order relevant tests and prescribe medication or recommend herbal/nutrient treatments when necessary. While a care team (for example, naturopath, acupuncturist, midwife and talk therapist) are the people you choose to trust to have your back, ultimately the hustle and grind that bring you good health are up to you.

However, there is a difference between knowing what normal blood pressure is for you and obsessing over the color of your pee. Be diligent and informed while also seeking balance. Just like you know that you can be trusted to make healthy choices, no approval needed, your body can be trusted to function, heal and use what you give it. If a problem arises, you can be trusted to address it or find the team that will help you manage that problem.

Girl, you got this.

Chapter Eleven

Guard the Door (For Your Other Half)

This chapter is for the other half of this baby equation. The emotion, bond and caring nature of so many dads and partners often moves me to tears. I realize that the other parent of a pregnancy is not always a man or the biological father of the baby. This chapter goes out to the hims, hers, theys and all the varieties of pregnancy partners. A pregnancy partner might also include the mother of the mother, the grandparents, the mother-in-law, the best friend, the sister, brother, or any other person who is invited to support this pregnancy and birth. This chapter is for you.

My first bit of advice: check your ego, amigo. I mean it. Bringing a child into the world is the ultimate humbling experience. Every baby is different. Every pregnancy is different. Every mother and every age is different. Remain humble and fascinated by the glory of your growing, changing life.

I hereby declare you, the guardian of this pregnancy. The best statement I ever heard from a dad was that it was his job to "guard the door." He determined who entered his wife's birth space and who was not allowed back. That particular dad did in fact guard the literal door, but there is also a figurative door here. While your pregnant sweetheart is an active participant in the health, flow and state of her life and this pregnancy, you are there for the overflow.

Help with the onslaught of questions and potential judgement from friends and family. Ask her best friend to take her for a mani-pedi because it's time!

In the rest of this book, I ask for accountability and ownership of your impact. Take action to reduce the stress you both feel. Life can be tremendously hard, and we're in this together so act like it. When your person's trauma comes knocking and she starts to spiral, guard the door. Pick her up; empower her. Here's a really crazy idea: you don't always have to know what to do. You can ask, "What can I do to help you?" Then really listen.

Your pregnant partner must be willing to link arms with you in this fight. They have to be willing to own their behavior too and admit when they've taken on too much or when their own bad habit is what is causing all this stress. You picked up this book because you are accountable, self-aware, ever changing, growing, evolving, humble, badass individual, and it's time to act like it.

While you are not the sun this pregnancy revolves around, you are deeply needed. Your love, attention, support, warmth, massages, kind gifts, middle of the night wakings, extra-large t-shirts and sweatpants are needed. Sometimes all you have to be is a witness. That lovely glowing pregnant goddess needs to be able to let go around you and vent without judgment. She needs to be able to say, "This sucks," and not be ashamed for not loving pregnancy. Sometimes she will even be mad at you. Remain humble, correct issues that are within your control and step back when you both need to cool off. Stay loving, patient and focused on the bigger picture.

Since Baby and your partner need you, they also need you at your best. That means good nutrition, exercise, plenty of water, self-care and balance. Self-care is not your permission slip to veg out on video games through all hours of the day and night. Carving out time for self-care is a struggle for every parent. Seek reasonable balance.

Some days you get to have some you-time while the baby takes an unexpectedly long nap and then you're wondering why the baby is sleeping so long. Some days you get three hours of sleep, and the baby does not want to be put down. You are partners in this, even if you are not a couple romantically. Help each other find the balance in the ways that work best for your individual situations.

I'm not here to be the couple's counselor, although I do suggest getting one even just for check-ins, but I cannot stress enough how important honest communication is. Communication is an important skill—if not the most important skill—in any relationship. I call communication a skill, because it's something many of us have to practice and develop, especially to do it effectively without gaslighting, manipulating, twisting words or projecting. It takes a lot to come to a conversation open, ready to listen and able to put all insecurities and predispositions aside, but it's worth it.

There is also a lot of value in hiring a mediator, even for an argument that most likely isn't going to be brought before a judge. I almost hired a mediator when my partner and I were trying to pick a name for our third son. Counseling, a trusted advisor and/or a mediator might seem like extreme measures, but they really aren't. We as people are not the same, and disagreements are inevitable; taking steps to solve those disagreements is often worth it. A neutral third party can work wonders.

I'm not going to include a list of things you can do, because the only person that should give you a list of what makes them feel loved and cared for is the person you are loving and caring for. With the right amount of commitment and humor, you can have conversations each time your needs as individuals change.

I'd like to take a moment to address dad fear. When you are in love and connected to a person, you feel their pain in your heart. You ache for them. When you watch your loved one in labor, that can bring up all sorts of feelings of helplessness, vulnerability and ache. It can even bring up trauma from previous births you've been part of. For a long time, I had the opinion that the birthing person should be the only one who decides where to give birth. I have had to chill a little bit on that opinion and come to the realization that the other half of the pregnancy matters too. If a husband is afraid that birthing at home could lead to a bad outcome, that feeling should be acknowledged and discussed. Is this fear based on evidence that is relevant to this pregnancy and this woman? Has he considered the benefit or his lady's desires? To a certain extent, decisions throughout the pregnancy should be a group decision, or at the very least, a discussion that is open and honest.

When you get to the birthing part, remain calm. I've been to births where the dad vomited, fainted, had an anxiety attack, got drunk, pushed me out of the way to catch his baby, cried, sat on his phone, leaped into the birth tub with her, forgot to put pants on, sat in the corner of the room with big deer-in-the-headlights eyes and held his wife lovingly as they welcomed their baby into the world. Pick which one you would like to do. If fainting doesn't sound optimal to you, then I recommend you eat and stay hydrated throughout labor and don't look if blood makes you lightheaded. Address your fear, watch birth videos, go to therapy, work through this before you are in the fetal position on the bathroom floor while your baby is being born!

I'm talking mostly to dads because these events are what my experience has been, but this could really apply to anyone. Silence your phone, address your fear and don't say stupid stuff. I attended a birth once where the mother-in-law to the birthing mother was talking on her phone. When she wasn't on her phone, her text notification was dinging over and over again.

She repeatedly asked me, "When do you cut the episiotomy?" (which I don't routinely do, by the way).

Her son told her to leave. I share this with you to remind you to prepare your team, especially if those planning to be at the birth have never been to a birth. The birthing space is sacred; treat it as such.

Chapter Twelve

The Third Trimester

H ere we are. I'm so glad you made it this far in this book! Oh, and in your pregnancy! I'm pretty sure there's a force in the universe that causes time to both speed up and slow down during pregnancy. You might find yourself saying "where did the time go?" and "when is it over?" in the same week. You're excited to meet your baby but also worried you won't get everything done before their arrival. You're ready to have your body back but nervous about birthing. I get it; it's a lot of mixed emotions. Just keep remembering, you got this. In fact, you were made for this.

Things you might enjoy (or not) during your third trimester: back pain, hip pain, joint pain, leg cramps, nausea, vomiting, heartburn, contractions (not just labor ones) and swelling extremities. Your baby may decide to produce an action movie starring your baby, co-starring the placenta and the cord. Your baby might spontaneously shake (this is not a scary seizure, I'll explain). You'll probably get tired of your partner making stupid comments, everyone asking you about the gender or the due date or if this is your first baby or are you scared for your vagina? (okay, maybe not that one, but people put their noses so far up in your business, we're just one generation away from this question, I think). And if it hasn't by now, your hair texture and thickness may change, your skin pigment may change, your fingernails and teeth sacrifice nutrients to your growing baby, even the consistency of your saliva changes. This is why we can say everything changes for our babies; literally our bodies morph into an entirely different being. You are now a mom.

Back pain, hip pain, and joint pain. I've already explained that your body is producing a hormone that relaxes your ligaments to make space for baby. I would have liked to have been a fly on the wall in the lab when the scientist who discovered this hormone named it.

"What shall I call this hormone that relaxes tissues? Hhhmmm, it relaxes stuff. Relax-about? Relaxing? No, too formal. Relaxin!"

Yep, it's called Relaxin. Brilliant minds at work here, people. Well, while your body is relaxin', it's also carrying extra weight, between your baby, the placenta and the extra fluid, there is additional strain on your muscles and joints. Things start to ache. While this is common, you shouldn't have to suffer and feel like that's just part of the deal. I do encourage you to seek care BUT seek care from professionals who know pregnancy and how to apply the appropriate techniques to a pregnant person. This includes massage, acupuncture, stretching and water aerobics. If you have previously enjoyed chiropractors, there are some practitioners who understand pregnancy and will do appropriate adjustments. Practice lifestyle habits such as avoiding prolonged periods of sitting or standing, taking healthy snack breaks at work, sipping water all day, and finding supplements that support you. Tools like the right clothes, a supportive belly band and a stability ball can also be helpful.

Calcium, magnesium and zinc are a trifecta of feel-good minerals. They help reduce cramping, relax and nourish muscles, strengthen your immune system and protect your bones and teeth. Find good food sources of these minerals and indulge. If you decide to supplement, do be aware that there are upper limits for everyone. Too much zinc at once will make you nauseous (and you've had enough of that), and too much magnesium will give you loose stool (or help move things along if you're backed up). Basically, spinach is your friend. Enjoy your salad.

If you birth vaginally, tears are a common concern. Your vagina and your perineal tissue are incredibly expansive. They can open and stretch to accommodate the width of your baby just as you and your baby were made for each other. Yes, those perineal stretching techniques you found on Pinterest can be helpful, although I no longer recommend using lavender oil because of the increase in synthetics that cause allergic reactions. I suggest warm castor oil, coconut oil, olive oil or simply your body's house lubricant (get it? like the house wine? *snickers*).

Whoever is catching your baby might say to you, "Breathe slow. Let your baby rest. Blow it out, not with a push."

This slowing down can allow the tissue to stretch rather than tear. The baby catcher can also apply gentle pressure to the perineum by placing the "swoop" of your flat hand at the base of your thumb on the perineum and protecting it. The goal is not to hold the baby in or apply any pressure to the baby but rather to guard the tissue itself. This hand position actually allows the baby to deliver over our hand. Lastly, you can place a warm washcloth on the perineum when pushing starts and as baby crowns. I recommend using whatever method of perineal protection the birthing person is most comfortable with, especially if this is the first vaginal birth or there is a history of tears.

Does anyone other than me find it tiresome how many things are named after male doctors? Braxton Hicks contractions were named after the gentleman who, well, decided to name them. He dubbed non-labor contractions Braxton Hicks in 1872, but we know women were having a nameless contraction long before he claimed them. Every woman and every pregnancy experiences these differently. Some women have reported feeling these as early as six weeks, but more often, they start poking at women during the third trimester. They can be painful, mild, intense, felt at the top or the bottom of the uterus or felt in your back or thighs. Think of it this way, when you go to the gym, you have to do one push-up before you can do ten, and you have to do ten before you can do one hundred. Your uterus is a muscle, and it requires training. You've been training it during your period—basically you're a bodybuilder on the inside. Your body knows the big task of birth is coming, and it knows what to do. These practice contractions can be caused by your movement, your baby's movement, someone touching your uterus, if you are startled, sneezing, coughing or laughing, dehydration, magnesium deficiency, if the wind blows or true labor. If you don't experience any labor drill contractions, don't worry, they might just be so mild you can't feel them, or your uterus is already saying, "I got this, Boo."

Sometimes a practice contraction happens all by itself. One rep and your uterus is all, "Screw this. Let's get ice cream."

Sometimes your uterus goes into beast mode. One contraction, then another, then another. They could be close together or not. One, two, three, your uterus is getting after it! It's like your uterus is listening to the hyped-up fitness instructor. "Okay, five more. You got this, let's go, and one, and that's right, eight more" (she tricks you every time).

This is called prodromal labor. The difference between it and true labor is that prodromal labor doesn't progress. The best thing you can do while your uterus is hitting those home workouts is take the opportunity to mentally prepare. Practice breathing through them, practice ignoring them, practice being in a positive mental state or repeat a mantra that feels good to you.

If you are more than thirty-seven weeks pregnant when this type of labor starts teasing you, drink water, have some tea and/or magnesium, lay down and chill. Breathe through it. If it's true labor, let it come. If it's training, thank it when it goes.

If you are not at least thirty-seven weeks pregnant call your care provider or go to the nearest emergency room. It could be premature labor, and you don't want to risk it.

Oh sure, breathing through your fifth round of prodromal labor while you chant, "I am not the least bit bothered by this," in that positive and graceful vibe while you sit on your lily pad would be lovely, but being at peace with it is not always going to happen. These contractions hurt. They suck, and being teased with the hope of labor starting can be frustrating. As usual, give yourself grace during this time and ask for what you need, whether that is more back massages or fewer projects at work. Remember, your baby can't stay in there forever.

I have often found the start-stop pattern of prodromal labor is due to the baby's position. I just imagine your uterus saying, "Hey, yous, let's move over this way." (I don't know why, in my head, your uterus sounds like a mobster—just go with it.)

Contractions don't simply move your baby down and out; they move your baby around too. Helping your baby get into an optimal position to manage the tight fit of the birth canal is one more magical way your body supports you and your baby in this pregnancy. Keeping that in mind, you can do things to help.

First, consult your care provider to determine what position your baby might be in. Maybe they are laying their back on your spine in a posterior position which makes it more difficult—although not impossible—for them to curve past your tail bone and pubic bone. Maybe your baby is looking at your back with her back to your front, but her head is tilted slightly to the side like she's confused about something (cue adorable puppy-tilting-head photo). Either way, you can help.

Your baby is sitting in water. If you move, that makes waves and encourages him to go with the flow. I highly recommend the website www.spinningbabies.com for techniques, poses and a thorough explanation of baby positions. Dancing is one of my favorite ways to love on babies from the outside. Move those hips, Mama, you sexy thang.

During my third pregnancy, I had so much prodromal labor for the weeks leading up to the actual birth, that I called my midwife and told her, if she made it stop, I would give her everything I own. I cried. I screamed. My partner was hiding sharp objects from me (too dark? Funny though). It's like it's designed to make us want to birth. At the beginning of pregnancy when the birth seems so far away, we can be afraid of it and wrestle with worries about it, but when it's the end and your uterus has become the most annoying Crossfit fanatic you've ever met, suddenly, you become ready. You find the strength to hope it comes and embrace the journey through birth.

Routinely, during the third trimester, some screenings are performed. Around twenty-eight weeks, your care provider might recommend you get a gestational diabetes test. If you've been pregnant before, you might remember this as the time you couldn't eat but had to drink a very sugary soda-thing then have your blood drawn an hour later.

This test is done because the symptoms of gestational diabetes are fatigue and frequent urination which, as you know, are also the foundation of pregnancy (and motherhood really). Pregnancy, by design, makes every woman insulin resistant, because the placenta needs to borrow some of her glucose (sugar/carbohydrates) for the baby's growth and development.

Normally, this is not a problem, but in some cases, this leads to excess sugar in your bloodstream. Best way to reduce the risk? What am I gonna say here? You know. I know you know. EAT RIGHT. If you don't overload your body with carbohydrates, then the excess sugar doesn't exist. I'm not taking away your every indulgence. There is nothing wrong with the occasional treat—I stress the occasional part. Every day is not occasional. Everything in moderation, Sis.

For this test, the drink you are asked to consume contains fifty grams of sugar, (there are also seventy-five and one-hundred-gram options) and if you are showing yourself all that veggies-, healthy fats- and protein-love, then fifty grams of sugar is a lot for your body, especially after fasting.

People with sedentary lifestyles with a poor diet and smokers are at the greatest risk for developing gestational diabetes. Family and personal history also play a part. Some providers due an initial one- or two-hour test and then ask you back for a more extensive assessment if your number is too high or too low. Other providers jump right into the three-hour testing, during which your blood is drawn multiple times over three hours. Sometimes gestational diabetes can be managed with diet, and other times, more help is necessary.

You can choose to not test at all. This is a risk assessment you and your trusted team can make together. You can choose the routine method, which is easy and can be compared with the results of many other women to establish a normal. You can choose to screen using a different form of sugar-loading, such as dextrose (the same sugar used in the lab glucose drinks) dissolved in water, a high carbohydrate/sugar meal (this is called postprandial screening) or many midwives have specific foods like candies that they have measured. Some women find using actual food helps them feel less nauseous and lightheaded, common side effects reported from the glucose drink.

You can also choose to do finger pokes and check your own blood sugar on a glucometer. This method can be valuable, because you learn how different foods affect your blood sugar, but it does involve some diligence and multiple finger sticks. Some of these methods are more evidence based than others, and some are still debated among peers. Medicine is ever changing, ever learning and sometimes staying the same way too long.

What if your care provider doesn't offer all these options? These are the options I offer my clients, but they aren't the only options either. Your care provider is there to make recommendations and advise you on the risks but not to make the decision for you. Midwives who attend births in homes or a birth center make risk versus benefits assessments on a regular basis. If the risk of a bad outcome exists, the midwife might recommend a hospital as a safer place to birth or a care provider who is better equipped to help the mother and baby. The ultimate goal is a safe birth, not a birth at a certain location.

Around thirty-five to thirty-eight weeks, you'll likely be asked if you'd like to do a GBS swab, or you won't be asked, and someone will just hand you a gown, tell you to lay back and stick a large q-tip up your vagina. Wait, what?

Rebel against this practice. They must ask and give you your options. GBS stands for Group B Streptococcus, a bacteria naturally occurring in your colon. Since your rectum and your vagina live awfully close to each other, GBS is like the neighborhood loud kids who run through everyone's front lawn. Sometimes GBS runs over to your vagina to play. Often the other flora and secretions of your vagina go out with a "get off my lawn!" (or rather "get off my bush!" is more accurate), and GBS clears out. Sometimes GBS gathers, and before you know it, they are having a party. This party is mildly annoying because GBS colonization is asymptomatic, and in most cases, doesn't cause any trouble. Many countries have stopped testing for GBS, because maternal to newborn transmission is so infrequent, and the results are not a definitive answer to the question "is my baby at risk?"

There have been cases of babies born to mothers who tested negative developing GBS infections, and there have been many cases of babies born to GBS positive mothers having no infection whatsoever. More research is needed for a more reliable predictor. In the US, GBS swabs are still routinely recommended. The United Kingdom stopped routine GBS testing in 2017, because the lack of assurance the test gives, the increased incidences of women getting antibiotics for no reason and the fact that most GBS-infected babies recover without complication. Given that information, many countries have decided not to test routinely.

If you test GBS-positive, you could test negative later that week or later that day! Your vaginal environment is everchanging, as it's supposed to be. It's designed to protect you from problems. There is no flaw in the system; it's not a mistake that our rectum and our vagina are neighbors. They know how to live next to each other and deal with each other's kids. However, like anything, GBS is not completely without risk. Newborn GBS infections do happen. The likelihood of an infection occurring depends on which study you reference, because the results vary. Some studies don't include data for mothers who didn't receive antibiotics during labor. GBS infections are the leading cause of meningitis. GBS colonization can increase the risk of chorioamnionitis, an infection of the amniotic fluid. It can increase the risk of your water breaking before you are actually in labor or before your baby is full-term. The current standard recommendation in the US is that a GBS-positive woman receive antibiotics through an IV during labor. Of course, antibiotics are also not without risk. The decision comes down to a risks versus benefits versus likelihood.

If you test negative, your provider might still routinely give you antibiotics during labor. They might not even tell you they are doing it. While I feel hospitals are moving toward more informed choice and less liberal use of antibiotics, I don't know if that is on a national scale. Just be aware you might not always be asked to exercise your right to choose, but you do still have that right. You can reduce the chances of GBS colonization by . . . what am I going to say here? You know . . . eat right, Queen! Your vaginal flora is affected by your gut flora so taking a probiotic can also be helpful. Vitamin C has an effect on regulating bacteria in general, however, there are no studies I'm aware of on the effect of vitamin C on GBS specifically.

You can decide not to test for GBS, or you can opt in. Some practitioners do the swab for you while you're on the table in the stir-ups (yee haw). At one point (and I'm not doing the research on where or how, because quite honestly, it's just not worth the time), practitioners were taught to swab the vagina then swipe or enter the rectum. Hold-up, does that make any sense? A bacteria naturally occurring in the rectum and a test that is looking for colonization of that bacteria in the vagina. Why would the swab belong near or in the rectum? Some practitioners still practice this technique, and they get a lot of positive GBS tests (I wonder why). Other practices send mothers to the bathroom with a swab and trust they know how to find their vagina. Not all care providers are familiar with the practice of mothers doing their own swab. Be prepared with your decision, and remember, it's your body, your choice.

Holy banana nut bread, you've done it. Your due date steadily approaches. I often get asked if nesting is really a thing—yes. You are biologically wired to prepare a safe space for your baby. Mama deer build a bed of grass where they will bed down and birth. Mama cats find a dark, secluded location. Nesting is natural, normal and good for the soul. De-clutter, feng shui, and Marie Kondo your home, car and office as much as you want. If anyone in your life, including yourself, is claiming you've lost it, kindly dismiss them; you have stuff to do.

Chapter Thirteen
La Placenta

Placentas are cool. I mean phenomenally awesome. Not only can you grow a whole human, but you can create an organ while laying on your couch. Queen, if that doesn't make you feel wildly capable, you need to check yourself. Your body is other-worldly. Think about it this way, from the very moment you were started in your mother's uterus, the universe conspired in your favor by using cells from the same cells that made you to create an organ which would act as the gateway for nutrients, oxygen and waste removal between you and your mother. Now it's happening again, in your body. This organ is the liver, kidneys, lungs, gut and endocrine system of a baby! Ah-mazing AF!

The placenta attaches to the wall of the uterus and uses brilliantly constructed vessels to transport products between the mother and baby without actually mixing maternal and fetal blood. It is the ultimate design of protection, preservation and love. There are some incidences when mother's and baby's blood mixes, and that is how we get early gender reveal blood tests, early genetic screenings, Rh sensitization and ABO incompatibility. These mixing moments are when the placenta first attaches and forms, and during birth. It can also happen if there is direct impact on the abdomen with significant force such as during a car accident, fall or other incidents. Sometimes these are acute and resolve; other times they require further action.

The placenta attachment site is an interesting topic because research has tried to figure out if there is a reason placentas attach in certain areas of the uterus versus other areas and if any of those attachment sites increase risk of certain outcomes. Here's what we know: a placenta over the cervix blocks the way for baby and means a surgical delivery is safer. An anterior placenta means the placenta is attached in the front. This makes it more difficult for you or your partner to feel baby move from the outside. If a placenta is attached to uterine scarring (such as from a cesarean section), this can increase the risk of complications, because it compromises the integrity of the scar tissue and the attachment of the placenta. Sometimes placentas favor certain locations because of the shape of the uterus, but we don't really know much else about why they do what they do.

For about the first ten weeks of pregnancy, your ovaries make progesterone, a hormone vital to the continuation of the pregnancy and partly responsible for how down you feel early on. From about ten weeks on, progesterone production is taken over by the placenta. This is also a system that helps reduce progesterone after birth to allow for the breastfeeding hormone prolactin to take over after the delivery of the placenta. Your body continues to be awesome.

In some cultures, placentas are sacred and carry part of the spirit of the baby. The practice of warming the placenta after birth if a baby is in distress came from this cultural belief and appears to hold at least some accuracy. Because of the deep connection the placenta has to the baby, practices like delayed cord clamping, lotus birth, cord burning and burying the placenta are common in these cultures.

From a Western perspective, we are more accustomed to the baby being born, dad cuts the cord within a few minutes, doctor gives a tug and out comes the placenta, which is quickly disposed of before the parents even know it existed. I cannot tell you how sad it is when I hear mothers tell me they didn't even know they had a placenta at their birth. Today, delayed cord clamping is defined in the Western obstetrician field as five minutes after the baby is born—five minutes!

Okay, sure, I've met cords that stop pulsing by five minutes, but the pulsing is not the only factor to consider here. Research tells us that even after the cord has stopped pulsing, stem cells are still migrating to the baby. Why not wait a little longer? Occasionally, it's necessary to cut a cord early, such as if there is an immediate medical concern and there is no time to get the placenta out to move it with the baby. Cords can be short or long. Sometimes they are too short to place the baby all the way up on your chest. Your baby might have to rest on your stomach or thigh until the placenta comes out.

There's also the convenience. Hospital staff are busy, overworked, understaffed and trying their best. No one has time to wait for your placenta or monitor the cord, and there's the whole we-don't-trust-patients part too. Through studies, we have also seen that if a baby needs to be resuscitated, the oxygen they get through the cord increases the chances of a successful resuscitation. I've heard the argument that babies need to be on the warmer for resuscitation. You know what was done before warmers? Babies were (and still are) resuscitated on their mother's chests or on a firm surface between her legs. The mother-baby unit is just that—one unit. Why would separation be a benefit to either of them? Unless that baby needs surgery or large equipment that can't be moved, everything can be done close to the mother. Did I get off on a little rant there? Okay, maybe.

Cutting the cord is that final physical separation of mother and baby. It should be acknowledged as significant and given its own time window. Not birth, clamp, cut, placenta, okay, we're done here. But instead: birth, mother and baby meet, bond, connect, placenta tucked in a bowl covered and placed close by. Then some talking, gender reveal, celebration, okay, let's cut that cord.

Lotus birth is when the cord is never cut. The placenta lives with the baby for the days after birth until the entire cord dries up and falls off. It's not as difficult as you might think, because the baby isn't exactly going hitchhiking and has to figure out how to pack his placenta. They stay in the same place, close to their person, breastfeeding, pooping, cooing and sleeping. The placenta is usually rubbed with salt and herbs, wrapped in absorbent pads and then a cloth for easy transport from the bed to the couch. The salt and herbs are partially traditional and assists with the drying, but mostly because the drying tissue can begin to smell unpleasant and pungent herbs can mask that a little.

Babies don't need a bath during this time, nor do they need to be passed around from person to person. Lotus birth encourages that mother-baby bond to stay intact in those days after birth which aids even further with that transition from inside to outside. Imagine living in one house your whole life. You have never left; everything you need has been provided for you. Suddenly that house starts tightening down, and even though it feels okay to go, once you step outside, you are exposed to completely new things. You risk sunburn, dry skin, sickness, bugs, dirt and loud noises. If you could just step out with another person who has been there before, if they would protect you, then you could grow to love this outside world. This other person makes it safe to keep going.

Some moms choose a partial lotus, when the placenta stays attached hours after birth—three, five, ten hours, however long until the mother feels ready. Typically, the cord is cut with a pair of special scissors, and a plastic clamp or special rubber bands are placed around the stump close to the baby's belly button. In regions where having sterile scissors is a luxury, lotus birth is more common or burning the cord takes place. This cauterizes the ends of the cord while separating placenta from baby. This method is slower, requires some extra precautions and leaves a longer stump because you don't want to burn too close to the baby. There is also often a startling pop as blood vessels burst in the heat. The slowness of it can feel more ceremonial and better at honoring that connection.

Some families bury the placenta with an object they believe will influence their baby's future, such as a book for intelligence, or a passed relative's item in hopes the baby will emulate that relative's character. Other families will bury it and plant a tree on top; as the baby grows, so does the tree. I planted a blueberry bush on top of one of my son's placenta and then watched while he ate the blueberries and played in the yard.

All mammals in the animal kingdom eat their placentas after

every birth, except humans. Taking a lesson from the animals, some women consume their placenta. At this point, I'm not sure I've heard it all, but I've certainly hear a lot. Women have cooked it like steak, blended it in smoothies, encapsulated it, eaten it raw (I picture Daenerys eating the heart on a platform surrounded by a chanting crowd), made a tincture, dried it and made tea and coated a piece in honey and swallowed it whole. This is a difficult thing to form studies on, because as you know, every woman is different, and every placenta is different. Without examining that particular placenta, running tests and potentially tainting it for consumption, we have no way of knowing what substances or foreign bodies are in that placenta.

We do know placentas carry hormones, one of which is oxytocin. A potential boost in oxytocin is often the focus when promoting the consumption of placentas. There is also progesterone, estrogen, testosterone and a myriad of other hormones in varying amounts. Whether or not those hormones maintain integrity under heat, cold and dehydration is unknown. We don't know how much of each hormone is in your placenta. Nor do we know how much potentially harmful bacteria is in it. Like other organ meats, placentas are rich in blood-building nutrients like iron, which a lot of women could at least use a little of postpartum. However, remember iron toxicity is a real thing.

Anecdotally, I've heard success stories and not so great stories about placenta consumption. It's a personal choice. I typically recommend, if you are planning to consume the placenta, please use safe, hygienic practices for processing, take small amounts at first and know your limits. I also recommend waiting until your milk comes in before consuming your placenta. I have seen early consumption delay the transition from colostrum to milk and that makes for a hungry baby.

One more note on consumption, if you choose lotus birth and your placenta has been sitting out for days at room temperature, then let's just think about that for a minute. Would you eat a raw steak that had been left out for days and had a certain unpleasant odor to it? No, at that point, your placenta is not safe either.

Consume, bury, burn, toss it or donate it to your local search and rescue for human remains practice searches with the dogs. What you do with your placenta is a very personal decision. If you are not too squeamish, I encourage you to look at it. Ask your care provider to explain it to you. Marvel in your ability to create a whole human and everything that human needed to survive in your womb. The vessels on a placenta often make a cool Tree of Life pattern. If you are believer, this can serve as a reminder of the imprint of God and how vast it is. If you take a more universe, all-that-is-just-is or scientific approach, then you can be fascinated by the natural brilliance of it. You can even ask for a print of your placenta on a piece of paper as a way to remember that connection between you and your baby.

Lastly, let's talk about how the placenta comes out. There's a pretty wide gap between care providers on how long they wait for a placenta to come out, so ask yours what their policy is and decide if that sits well with you or not. Once your baby is born, the placenta starts shunting blood and nutrients to the baby. The placenta then peels away from the uterine wall. Sometimes it starts in the middle, causing blood to pool behind it. Once an edge separates, there may be a small gush of blood known as the separation gush; it's normal and quickly over.

Other times, the bleeding is in lower quantities but lasts longer. This just means the placenta started separating from the edge, and there was no pool of blood to gush. If your placenta is allowed to take its time, your body works with its natural clotting factors, and the contractions of your uterus tighten around this new internal wound and stop the bleeding. If the placenta is rushed out, clotting factors and your uterus have to catch up, sometimes causing extra bleeding.

Now, I have seen babies come quickly, and the placenta rolls out right on the baby's heel. That's just the way that body decided to do things. Sometimes the uterus needs help to catch up. Ask yourself, do you trust your care provider to tell you when you placenta has to come out or when that extra help is necessary? Do you suspect your care provider would rush the placenta? Is your body fortified with nutrients to give your uterus the energy it needs and your blood the nutrients it needs to save your life?

I have one bit of not-so-great news: the contractions continue after birth. Sorry, Mama. Your uterus continues to contract to deliver your placenta, tighten over the placenta wound to stop bleeding, to expel fluid and membranes to prevent infection, and to start the process of returning you to your pre-pregnancy state. These can feel like really awful period cramps, or they can be mild, but they are necessary.

Breastfeeding produces oxytocin which causes more contractions. You've been warned. This is by design. Breastfeeding produces that feel-good-bonding hormone to help you connect with and nurture your baby, while it also works to conserve your energy by reducing your blood loss and putting your uterus back where it was. Oxytocin loves you.

I could ramble on for days about this, but I promised you a basic summary. I hope you share in my gratitude for placentas and the cascade of hormones that work to protect you and your baby. Whatever you choose regarding the management of the cord, when to cut it, and what to do with your placenta after do your own research.

Chapter Fourteen

Labor

You've been waiting, planning and prepping. You're so ready! There is a lot to say about labor and birth; it seems to be the topic on everyone's lips in conversations about pregnancy. Birth can even be political and spur many heated conversations in moms' groups (especially from Judgey Mc-cranky Pants).

We aren't here to debate the politics on women's bodies or the pressure from insurance companies driving medical policies and protocols. I will, however, make this rant: I am so fed up with women who have desires being called divas, bitches, snobby, picky and basic. Knowing what we want makes us self-aware, self-loving and in control of healthy boundaries. Not only does getting our preferences met make us feel good and improve our overall demeanor, it also improves our relationships, our health and our distinctive lives.

When our preferences are met, we are happier, feel safer and more able to flow in our purpose. This is never truer than in birth. You are absolutely worthy of being touched, talked to, respected and provided for in the manner in which you prefer throughout your entire labor, birth, and quite honestly, your life. If anyone on your support team or birth team doesn't get that, they can bounce. In fact, it's officially your partner's job to bounce them.

Okay, but what if you can't voice what you want? You're focused and working your way through contractions. You don't have the words to ask your doula to massage your back or ask your husband to get out of your face. This is one reason that conversations with your team beforehand are important. Helping your team get to know your preferences will enable them to read your mind a little while you're in labor. Sometimes our preferences change in labor. You might normally like when your husband rubs your feet but now is not the time! That's okay too.

Plan a single word with your team that can mean whatever you want it to. Maybe butter means "stop touching me" and balls! means "I'd like an epidural please." There is huge value in a person in the room being able to read you. Whether that means an annoyed look at your partner is interpreted as he better get his sister out of the room before she posts your birth on social media or a pleading look at your doula that let's her know you need extra support 'cause this is getting real.

Have those conversations, set your boundaries and stand by them. Some boundaries you set might include:

- No one posts your birth on social media without your permission
- Only the people you select are allowed in your birthing space
- No one holds your baby before you
- Everyone must have their phones on silent
- Certain smells are not allowed in your space
- Your favorite postpartum food is in the fridge, and if anyone eats it, they will be force fed laxatives until all your food and then some is out of their system
- No one is to bother you for an update if you've gone past your due date. "Thank you all for your concern. The baby and I are healthy. We will update you when there is a change."

Sit down and write out your desires but be aware that labor and birth are fluid. Leave room to flow and surrender to the labor this baby will bring you.

I'd like to take a moment in this chapter to discuss VBAC, which stands for vaginal birth after cesarean. VBAC is something a majority of women who have experienced a C-section can attempt; however, many care providers are still using fear-based tactics to convince people to get repeat C-sections. Cesarean sections are major surgeries and should be recommended sparingly. One of the arguments in favor of the repeat C-section is the increased risk of uterine rupture. Uterine rupture is a serious, life-threatening event that is rare—we're talking less than 1 percent by multiple studies. C-sections are not without risk, including increased risk of hemorrhage, blood clots, amniotic fluid embolism, risks of future complications with pregnancies, infection, longer recovery time and reactions to anesthesia.

Is a repeat C-section the best thing for you and your baby? Are you approaching the decision with fear? What about with adequate information? I don't deny that C-sections can be necessary. We are fortunate to live in a time when these surgeries are performed by highly trained doctors under conditions that make C-sections much safer than they were in the first half of the twentieth century. What I'm concerned about is a lack of complete transparency.

Does uterine scarring increase the risk of uterine rupture? Yes, by a fraction of a percent.

Is there a risk of rupture even if you've never had a C-section? Yes, also rare. This goes back to making risk versus benefits decisions, which we do every day. We choose, daily, to accept risks that we feel are worth it. I encourage you to assess the risk relevant to your individual situation if you are considering VBAC versus cesarean.

A due date is not a birth date—it marks forty weeks of pregnancy. About only 5 percent of babies are born on their due date, and that's assuming the due date is correct. After thirty-seven weeks gestation, a pregnancy is considered full term. After thirty-seven weeks, the risk of complications due to premature labor and birth are significantly reduced (whew!). In most states where CPMs and LMs are regulated, home birth attended by your local midwife is an option after thirty-seven weeks for healthy, low-risk pregnancies.

Your due date is like ordering something online and seeing the date it will arrive in bold letters on the screen. It's coming on that day. That's the day you'll tear open the box and get the thing you've been waiting for! The day arrives. There it is—the box on your front porch, but instead of the baby you've been waiting for, it's three Braxton-Hicks contractions and some heartburn. You check your email and see the ever-daunting message, "Your order has been delayed. Sorry for any inconvenience." You are inconvenienced, and that due date can kiss your ass.

How far you go past your due date is between you, your baby and your care provider. You might be monitored a little more closely with extra appointments, an additional ultrasound or two and/or extended periods of time listening to your baby's heartrate. These are all just precautionary measures to make sure your baby is handling the extra time inside well, which they often do. "You've been pregnant for x weeks," alone is NOT a reason to induce your labor or perform a C-section.

The concern with babies who kick back and relax on the inside past the due date is that the placenta could "age out" and become less efficient until it is no longer adequately supporting your baby. While this is possible, it's not so common that we need to jump to forcing labor and risk the side effects from doing so. Again, all of life is a risk versus benefits assessment and gives you very personal decisions to make. Make decisions from an informed, empowered place (Is there an echo in here?).

What usually happens is your placenta releases chemicals that tell your body, "Okay, we're ready now," and so the cascade of hormones that start and carry labor through birth and postpartum begin. If labor does not start naturally for you, there is nothing wrong with you. I truly believe in the deep parts of my soul that we are protected by the universe (or G-d, higher power, whatever you believe), and how our babies come into the world shapes us and them in exactly the way it was meant to.

I wish I could tell the families I serve exactly how labor starts, when labor starts and how it will progress, but honestly, that would ruin the unique adventure that labor and birth is. It's a monumental event. Let's discuss some possible signs of labor and maybe debunk some things you've heard.

Losing your mucus plug does not mean you're going into labor. First of all, calling it a plug is a little deceiving. It's not a cork like on a wine bottle. If it was, my practice might see more women doing questionable things with wine openers (for the record, those don't belong in your vagina—don't). It's just mucus, a protective barrier over your cervix that begins to shed at the end of pregnancy. It can regrow and shed again, or you may not notice it at all. It can be sticky, gooey, white or clear, and it kind of looks like your vagina sneezed in your underwear.

The old, standard, 5-1-1 rule was that you call your midwife or go to the hospital when your contractions were five minutes apart and one minute long for one hour. This rule has proven to be inaccurate and, in some cases, unsafe. Let me be clear: your body, your uterus, your baby and your pregnancy ARE UNIQUE, which means your labor is unique. Some women start labor with contractions three minutes apart; some women go from twenty minutes apart to two minutes pretty quickly. Some people never get any closer than eight minutes apart. These are examples of normal labor that don't fit the designated rules of labor. The unpredictability of labor is one of the tricky things about it, and one of the reasons some people barely make it to the hospital or birth center or don't at all. Labor is unpredictable. I don't say this to scare you; I say this to inform you. Trust your instincts and make those false alarm calls/visits if necessary. You may be experiencing prodromal labor, but at least you'll be checked on, and the contractions will fade and leave you alone. Contractions may be felt in the top, the side or the bottom of the belly, the low back and your thighs.

Diarrhea or loose stool can be a sign that your body is preparing for labor. It's not often a sign that labor has started nor is it an absolute sign of labor. Sometimes it just means you ate some bad chicken. Anytime someone sees blood, it can be alarming (don't ask me why I'm putting diarrhea and blood in the same paragraph; it's my book and I do what I want). We are taught that blood outside our bodies means danger. In reference to blood as a labor sign, some spotting can be normal. As the cervix dilates, the vessels that feed it bleed a little. This blood should be bright red to pink and in small amounts. Dark red or heavy bleeding is concerning; seek immediate help.

It seems like a lot of people believe that labor has begun when the mother and everyone around her are standing in a puddle of water. Your baby, placenta and all the amniotic fluid is held within a double layered membrane sac. The water breaking is when both layers pop a hole and release some of the amniotic fluid. Often this happens during labor, after contractions have started and sometimes even just before the baby is seen. Sometimes the membranes rupture, and labor doesn't start right away. Typically, in a case like this, labor starts within hours. Once the membranes are confirmed ruptured, there is a slight increased risk of infection because that protection barrier has a hole in it. This means, if you suspect your membranes have ruptured, do not put anything in your vagina. I know, I never let you do anything fun. Don't take a bath, douche or engage in physical activity that causes you to sweat. Put on some breathable underwear and a pad, call your care provider and trust that everything will be fine.

Other signs of labor may include rectal pressure, feeling restless with a sudden burst of energy, nausea, vomiting, leg cramps, sudden emotional shift, sudden anger outburst and your intuitive knowing. Labor is a fickle bitch. She comes and goes. She teases you. Sometimes she shows up with a vengeance; sometimes she sneaks in and sits down without you even noticing. Next thing you know, you're pushing! These signs are not definitive signals you are in labor (although the baby head between your legs would be a definite yes, you're in labor), but they are things you should report to your midwife.

At the forefront of every pregnant woman's mind is "will I be able to handle the pain?" The short answer is, yes, you can handle anything. Just in case you aren't feeling powerful, co-creator vibes during your tenth hour of labor, I'll talk about some drug-fee ways to cope.

A favorite coping tool of mine is water. Have you ever noticed that water is quite central to our lives? We are created in it, washed in it and baptized in it. The water inside us rocks toward the moon and flows back to the earth in a sequence so eloquently known to our souls. We are grown in water, then washed into mothers with this water. Our creation centers are cleansed of anything that might have happened there before each birth. Considering how vital water is to our lives, it makes sense that many women feel drawn to birthing in the water.

Water birth is becoming increasingly more well known, thank goodness! Because of the additional considerations, I recommend only birthing in water with a trained attendant. As those labor waves rush through your body, sinking into a warm pool of water can help ease the tension in your muscles just enough to bring your pain from a 10 to a 9.5. If you are someone who typically enjoys a bath for relaxation, then a birth tub will likely also feel soothing to you. If baths are not your thing, a warm shower can still do wonders to help you feel more comfortable.

A few things to consider about laboring and birthing in water: with birth comes poop, blood, amniotic fluid, urine and sometimes even baby poop. All of that will be floating around the tub with you. Once you've had a baby, you don't even notice what color the water is in your tub, but some women would really prefer not to sit in that.

For your baby to safely birth into the tub, the water temperature must not be so cold that it stimulates her to take a breath and inhale water. Between 98 and 100 is the perfect temperature. That's a toasty tub that can cause you to feel uncomfortably warm and dehydrate quickly.

Laboring in the tub over an extended period will result in your tub temperature dropping. Do you remember the old timey movies when a woman goes into labor and someone says, "Boil some water"? I still get to say that, though less dramatically. Adding pots of hot water to your tub will help it maintain temperature. Your care team will also recommend breaks from the tub to decrease the risk of dehydration.

You'll need certain equipment for a water birth: towels, towels and towels. It's likely you will be in and out of your tub more than once. Multiple towels to dry you and your baby off quickly will be needed.

You can purchase a tub designed specifically for birthing. They have high sturdy walls, inflate into many different rooms in your home, have room for you to change positions comfortably, and can often fit two people (or three after the baby arrives). You'll need a brand-new hose designed for drinking water only (garden hoses may contain chemicals), an adapter to connect the hose to the water source and a birth pool liner usually available by the manufacturer of your birth pool. Try out your adapter before you are in labor, because no one is going to the hardware store at two in the morning to get a new one.

I have attended births in some household tubs, but there is strict criteria for that. Tubs must be clean. I recommend against jetted tubs because it is very difficult to guarantee the interior of the jets is free of bacteria. Your baby's new immune system is too delicate to risk exposure to festering bacteria at birth. Your bathroom should also be big enough to fit your whole team, your partner, the midwife, doula, midwife's assistant, photographer—it can get tight.

When birthing anywhere in your home, your midwife will assess how easily an emergency medical crew could get to you if necessary. If you are birthing on your third floor up a spiral staircase, you may want to reconsider.

There are a lot of options for ways to birth or ways to get through labor. What it really comes down to is what do you want? Personally, I never got into the deep breathing and meditating through labor and birth. I screamed my babies out. I mean, I woke the dead, and I still consider my births beautiful, enlightened and life changing. Part of that is I had the right team. My midwives remained calm and trusted my ability to voice when I needed something else. If meditation, silence, low moans, deep breathing, prayer or any other safe technique feels good to you, then that is exactly what you should do. If you like sound therapy, sounds or moans in a low tone may help move your energy downward.

You should be allowed to scream without people asking if you are okay and if you want an epidural every twenty minutes. You should also be able to labor in a quiet, dark room while no one talks to you or touches you. How the system should work is that you say something like, "I'm thirsty," and water magically appears in the hands of your doula who is putting the straw in your mouth. You should be able to say, "Something feels wrong," and your team of birth workers jump into action to determine what could be wrong and work to fix it.

A note to people of color: I SEE you. I hear as you sit across from me and tell me you're afraid the white doctor will ignore you. I hear your fears that you won't be believed when you say something is wrong. I'm listening; tell me how to best care for you. I hear from my patients of all skin colors that they felt something was off and their care provider dismissed them. I see these deep generational wounds. I see women who believe that their bodies are not capable and doubt their worthiness to speak up. I watch them trust hospitals, systems and protocols that let them down over and over again.

You have choices, these are your rights! You are worthy of good, attentive, informed and respectful care! Many women are here healing, pushing back and rising up. Sometimes it feels like a lonely journey, but we're here. I offer you a big, written hug and say, I know it's hard, Baby. Keep going.

Unfortunately, labor is not always what we hoped and imagined it would be. Sometimes there is a complication that changes the course your labor travels. No matter how it twists and turns, I hope you feel respected and empowered.

The birth tub is often referred to as the midwife's epidural. Since home birth midwives don't administer epidurals or pain medications, we work with the body's natural, feel-good methods. Besides water and vocalization, some other options for pain management include distraction, massage, music, heat, movement, a make-out session (with your partner—not your midwife), laughter and a positive mental attitude.

Because I value my life, I have never told a woman in labor that she should think positively. Instead, I give specific ideas to focus on:

- This won't last forever
- One contraction at a time
- There's a baby at the end of this
- Your body was made to do this
- Billions of women have done this before you
- You can have *insert favorite dessert* when you're done

Maybe from now on I will recommend women read my book when they go into labor, and they will be instilled with all the positive vibes and empowerment I have to offer.

Relax your holes. The best advice I can give any woman in labor is relax your holes. Your body is connected through the intertwined nerves, vessels, muscles, fascia, fluid and energy that flow throughout. During labor, clenching your jaw and biting down is counterproductive to relaxing and opening your vagina. Relax your holes. Your tongue hole, your bathroom hole (which is lady speak for rectum) and your baby hole.

Do it right now, while you're reading. Relax your face; feel the muscles by your ears down to your throat go soft. Take a deep breath. Let your breath move down through your body as if you are breathing out of your vagina. Feel your pelvic floor let go. Shift your weight and be aware of your glute muscles. They are round and perfect, 'cause, girl, you've got it going on. Now relax them. Picture the wave of relaxation flowing down your low back through your glutes and into your thighs.

Revisit this practice of relaxing your holes on a regular basis and especially during labor. If you're having a hard time softening your lips and mouth during labor, kiss someone. Someone you've been given permission to kiss, like, warn your doula if you're going for it. You can also blow through your lips like you are motor boating some double Ds or making a sound like a horse pushing air out—a majestic horse with perfect hair.

Labor is the last mile of a marathon, the one-hundredth rep of squats, the 300th day of being stranded on a deserted island, and you finally see a ship in the distance with your baby on it, but why isn't it coming faster? It's a mother fucking feat, y'all. No matter how your labor plays out, you are the only one who went through it. Others may drive the golf cart alongside you, but you are running the whole thing. There comes a moment when you—a human with a uterus— can either fight what your body was made for or surrender.

Surrender to the hormones that came into existence for this purpose. Surrender to the fear. Give up all the preconditioned ideas about what labor and birth should be. Surrender to what it is. Surrender to what you get to decide it is—a demonstration of one of your body's most wildly wonderful capabilities. Whoa, you can pass a person through your bones and supply them with all the oxygen they need to make the journey via an organ that you created, while hormones not only guide the baby out but also support you, your baby and your body through surviving and loving the whole thing. G-d is good.

Chapter Fifteen
What Else Comes Out of Your Body?

I understand that women don't want to poop during birth. It's not the most lady-like thing we could ever do, but this is why you shouldn't invite anyone to your birth that you wouldn't poop in front of. Sphincters are pretty socially awkward, and if your rectum won't open to empty your bowels, then you just end up with more stuff crammed into a tiny space.

Don't be a pelvic hoarder; pee and poop to make room for your baby. Most likely, you won't be able to help it. If there is poop in there, it will be squeezed out like a toothpaste in a tube as your baby moves down. So really, it's a good sign that your baby is moving down. Yea, poop! You may not even notice. Your care provider might gently wipe your butt (because that's love) and toss the tissue before you can say "what's that smell?" and your care provider says your partner's name with shock and disgust (again, out of love). Then your team will forever pretend that your partner fluffed, and you were a perfect lady.

Spotting or blood-tinged toilet paper when you wipe is normal. If you are not pushing or actively birthing your baby and placenta, then a flow of blood or anything roughly over a tablespoon could be a sign of a problem; seek help.

The blood that happens during birth comes from two places: (1) from the south where your cervix is dilating, and any scratches or tears can bleed, and (2) north of that where your placenta was implanted. Once the placenta separates from the lining of the uterus, it leaves an open wound. As your uterus shrinks, the area bleeds less and less until it heals.

When there is too much blood, it's called a hemorrhage. This is a common concern for families. Try to remember, some bleeding is normal, and your body can handle it. Also remember, to the untrained eye, the bleeding from birth can look like a lot but actually be a very underwhelming amount to the care provider. Another thing to note is the amniotic fluid in there with the baby can sometimes add to the blood, making it look like more.

When there is more blood loss than your body can handle, that is a postpartum hemorrhage. You have trusted yourself to pick your team, and this is one of the cases in which your team will step up and help your body stop bleeding, so you can regain strength.

"She threw up." This is often the call I get from dads in the middle of the night, and my usual response is, "Oh fun! What else is she doing?"

Basically, when labor starts, the human body expels everything. If it's mobile, it might come out. This applies to food, fecal matter and your baby. The uterus is made up of muscle fibers that run in multiple directions. It's incredibly strong and happens to sit right next to your stomach, intestines and bowels. The pressure from your uterus can cause that upchuck reaction. For most women, it doesn't last the whole labor, and for those that it does, there is an end eventually. If vomiting in labor continues for a long time, there are concerns about dehydration that your birth team will address with you. It should look something like this:

Care provider: "Hey, you've been throwing up for five hours now, and I'm concerned about dehydration. Would you mind if we place an IV to help with that? It would be a solution of salts and sugars that may make you feel less nauseous. Are you okay with that?"

You: Sweating and nodding.

or

You: "I really hate needles. Is there another option?"

Care provider: "If you can drink these rehydration solutions and keep them down for about an hour, that could be helpful."

You: "I'll try the drink."

THAT is informed and respectful care. If in that scenario, you, your uterus or your baby started to show signs of dehydration, your care provider will likely revisit the IV. It's still your choice, but you have to be ready to accept the consequences of your choices—good and bad. That's just life.

Let's talk about amniotic fluid. This is the fluid your baby swims in for months. Amniotic fluid is basically a really fancy, electrolyte drink. It's usually clear, unless your baby poops in it, which then makes your uterus a fishbowl while your baby just swims around in their own poop. Cute little guppy, though. Amniotic fluid is mostly water with some minerals, peptides and carbohydrates. If you are dehydrated, there is less water available for your amniotic fluid. Dehydration can also cause unnecessary contractions, so drink-up.

I cannot emphasize enough how important it is to keep your bladder empty during labor. Your bladder lives next door to your uterus. If it's full, then your bladder will be leaning over and pushing on your uterus. This intrusion can decrease the intensity of contractions, make it more difficult for your baby to come down and make you less comfortable as your bladder and your baby compete for space. Your bladder can also trap your placenta, like when you're trying to go somewhere and your neighbor stops you in the driveway for a chat. Most concerning is when your bladder is just full enough to keep your uterus from continuing to shrink after the birth of your placenta. Continuing to contract and shrink is how your uterus stops you from bleeding out of your placenta site. If the uterus can't shrink, the bleeding can't stop.

Your bladder doesn't have to be at max capacity to cause continuous bleeding. Get your bladder out of the way. If someone at the hospital has placed a urinary catheter for you, then that's one less thing for you to think about. If you are laboring without a catheter and getting to the toilet sounds impossible, ask your team for an absorbent pad or other option so you can urinate. If you start to bleed excessively, your midwife might use a urinary catheter to get your bladder out of the way. If this is something you are adamantly against, discuss it ahead of time.

If you pee, poop, puke, sweat or bleed, nutrients are leaving your body. Labor snacks should be things you like to eat. Now is not the time for kale chips. You want food easy to digest with a quick sugar boost. Some of my favorites are a spoon full of honey, bananas, any berries, half a piece of toast with jam or honey, and fruit leather.

I talk about what to eat after birth in the postpartum chapter. During labor, sipping on water, an electrolyte drink, a vitamin C drink or red raspberry leaf tea will also help you maintain energy and effective contractions. I am referring to out-of-hospital births; hospitals have their own policies on what you can eat or drink while in labor. Ask your care provider about this ahead of time, so you can be prepared.

Chapter Sixteen

D is for Delivery

How dilated am I!?!?!"
"How dilated is she?"

Somewhere along the development of birth, someone decided that cervical dilation was the only thing that would determine how soon the baby was coming, how much progress a person has made and what the next step should be. I am here to tell you, your cervix is none of anyone's business. You, my love, have made a huge amount of progress. Centimeters don't define your progress.

The standard assessment today is one centimeter per hour equates to appropriate progress. Any longer than that, and some providers are taught to be concerned. Your cervix is not a measuring stick for labor. Your cervix does not have to open in any certain amount of time. In fact, it's quite common for women to walk around with a three-to-four-centimeter dilated cervix. Don't you feel the breeze? Women can jump from four centimeters to seven in less than a couple hours, or they can sit at six centimeters while laboring for eight hours, especially if they are stressed.

Do you love my analogies yet? Okay, recap. Due dates are like Amazon packages, labor is a marathon, husbands are nightclub bouncers and a cervix is like a cat (no relation to pussy . . . okay, a little). Your cervix wants to lay around, all tucked up next to your baby for months until it just wants to come forward, open up and let your baby pass by. Your cervix will come along and rub against your leg all friendly like; here comes another cozy contraction, so it opens up to you a little more. But then someone reaches out to pet the cervix. "What the Frisky do you think you're trying! I did not say you could TOUCH me!" It's a fickle kitty.

Now, if the cervix is a cat, then oxytocin is catnip. Oxytocin is the love hormone. It causes contractions, bonds us to our partners, bonds us to our babies and makes us feel all warm and fuzzy. Some things that raise oxytocin levels are seeing baby animals (OMG puppies!), watching others birth blissfully, kissing, hugging, sex, meditation, touching, saying "I love you" or other loving statements (like "I made coffee"), cuddling, singing, music, dancing and petting an animal. Makes sense, right? Those things feel really good with the right person/people.

You know what doesn't increase oxytocin? Bright lights, chatty nurses, beeping machines and gloved hands up your vagina (unless you're into that—no judgment). When I enter the home of a laboring woman, I sneak in and sprinkle catnip all over the place. I turn on the soft music, turn down the lights, make it warm, make it safe, and if I must, send the husband in topless! (Makes birth with me sound like a late-night show. I am a professional, I promise.) I usually leave the cervix alone. I'm more interested in what the baby is doing. How is Baby's heart rate? Is Baby moving? What is Baby's position? These are the things I assess throughout labor.

Especially if this is your first birth or first vaginal birth, one thing that can stall delivery is anterior lip. Anterior is an anatomical direction referencing the front of the body. So, an anterior lip is a small, lip-sized (like the ones on your face) portion of your cervix at the front—or top if you're laying down on your back. Usually this means Baby needs to adjust their head and put a little more pressure on this part of the cervix, which often happens naturally. If a mom changes positions and helps Baby move, that will help apply that pressure. "Moving moms moves babies," I can hear my preceptor in my head.

An anterior lip can slow labor and exhaust moms because they get frustrated not understanding what's going on. If I suspect an anterior lip is holding things up, I might do an exam to confirm it but not always. Then we talk through ways to resolve it.

Besides a stall in labor, the only other reason I might do a vaginal exam doesn't have anything to do with the cervix; it has to do with signs that the baby is not coming with the head or butt first. If a baby is offering up a foot, hand, shoulder, hip, back etc., I would quite like to know. Please pause here and tell your baby not to pull that shenanigan.

When a baby advances sideways into the birth canal, it's called malpositioned or malpresentation. A baby cannot be born vaginally sideways. This doesn't happen often. If your baby is not engaged in your pelvis, he can often adjust his position before labor begins, but if you're in active labor and your baby is trying to wave at you through your vagina, a hospital is the safest place for you and your baby to be. Once your home birth midwife recognizes this, she will help you get to the hospital the safest way possible. Your body and your baby are very smart, and a malpresentation will often show signs like inconsistent contractions or stalled labor.

Your midwife can use her skilled hands to feel your belly and assess what position your baby is in at the appointments leading up to labor and in early labor. Keep in mind, while your midwife does what she can to identify malpresentation, we don't have x-ray vision and are sometimes surprised. In these surprise scenarios, we are trained to act quickly and make the safety of you and your baby our top priority.

While we're on the topic, let's talk breech. Babies can be born breech. Babies have been born breech. With a breech-trained provider, breech birth can be safe, beautiful and really freaking cool. The trick is having a knowledgeable provider who is trained in the special consideration for breech birth. Breech presentation alone is not a reason for a C-section. If there are other risk factors or if the provider you want is not trained in breech, then you might not be having a vaginal birth discussion anymore. The choice is yours; just be informed and aware of the reasons for provider recommendations.

Okay, you've gotten through pregnancy, you've ignored early

labor until you can't anymore, you've taken deep breaths, kept your bladder empty and rocked your hips through active labor . . . it's time. You feel heavy pressure in your rectum, maybe a widening feeling very low in your pelvis and pressure down on your pelvic floor. Let this come. Trust that your body and your baby know the way, breathe and make a low moan that pulls all of your focus down. You can't help it; your body pushes for you. Your baby often rocks down and then back up just a little, which allows all that tissue to stretch, your baby's head to mold and the whole world to open up. Cheese grits, I love my job! Sometimes, it's called for to give a push and help baby out or help move things along. Your experienced midwife is trained to know when to ask you to do that.

If this is your first vaginal birth, you may feel that low pressure and think it's time to start pushing with everything you have. This often leads to an anterior lip, a tired and frustrated mom, and a confused partner. Let the pressure build, let the sensations come; surrender, my love. You got this.

Once you dilate to twelve centimeters, (Yes, I know there is only ten, but we've established that you're an overachiever) the next sensations feel big, this is what you've been waiting for. Your baby will rock down and back up a little as she moves through your bones and stretches your tissues out and then suddenly, "Oooooooo, that burns!"

That is your baby with a full crown out of your body and stretching your perineum, the tissue along the bottom of your vaginal opening. It's very stretchy and totally made for this. Your baby might crown and slide back in a little. Pause there and let your perineum adjust to the change or your baby might keep going fast and hard. None of these are wrong, each of these has things to consider.

1) Your baby slides back in a little. This can be totally normal, and on the next contraction, your baby usually comes out quite a bit further than the last time OR this can be a sign that Baby is trying to reposition a shoulder and may need some assistance. As a midwife, I gently use my hands to assist your baby, making enough space and positioning his shoulder properly for delivery. I can't tell you what

another care provider would do or what tool they would use, because it's largely based on skill, comfort and the education they received.

2) Your baby pauses. This can feel really intense, like someone trying to kidnap you by pulling on your ear but you refuse to go. If you can focus on your breathing and make slow but short inhales and exhales while holding your baby there, that is ideal. Let the tissue stretch, picture yourself walking on a beach, glare at your husband and try not to panic. This will greatly reduce your chances of tearing. This is also usually the time when dads say some cuss words. Try to keep your cool, Dad.

3) Baby comes hard and fast. Often when babies come fast, it's because Baby's position is all lined up, and no adjustments are necessary. Your contractions are strong AF, and that is just the birth you were both meant for. Sometimes, because the tissue didn't have time to stretch, there is tearing. Don't worry, you will heal. Sometimes a quick birth was made possible because your baby was a little smaller, and this makes tearing less likely. Babies who come fast often start breathing without any problem. Occasionally, Baby takes a moment before they breathe when birth is fast, because they were just inside your warm body, and now they are in the lights, smells, sounds and temperatures of the outside. It's a big change; they need a moment.

Let's talk more about those fast births. When I hear women say, "I just hope it's a fast labor," I remind families that fast births come with their own caveats. Birth is a big event and happening really fast can make it feel even bigger. It can even leave the mother and her partner in a moment of shock. Focus on the priorities. The baby needs to breathe. The mother needs to connect with her baby. The uterus needs to contract down to a smaller size to stop bleeding.

If your labor is progressing quickly, the best you can do is ground yourself—feel your hands, feel your feet. Breathe. Find a point to focus on. During the birth of my fourth child, I found myself locking eyes with the Pikachu on my middle child's pillowcase. Hey, whatever works. Be as present as possible.

Immediately after a fast birth, everything needs time to catch up, and your baby and your uterus sometimes need help. Helping your baby can look like rubbing your baby, changing your baby's position, suctioning your baby's mouth and nose with a rubber bulb, or using a bag and mask to inflate your baby's lungs.

If your uterus needs some help, someone in your birth team will likely rub the top of your uterus with a hand on your belly. The stimulation from the rubbing helps your uterus contract and tighten down to stop any bleeding. Your team might also encourage your placenta to come and/or help you find a way to empty your bladder.

After crowning, your baby's head slides out, lubricated by nature itself. Once your baby delivers out to his/her chin (like a warm, cheesy pizza), you suddenly find yourself in a room of people staring at your vagina. It's beautiful. Because your baby's neck is narrower than its head, you may feel a relief of the pressure on your perineum, but this is also the moment when your baby turns their head and might wiggle their body, so you trade one sensation for another.

Let's pause here. It's a common fear that the umbilical cord will be wrapped around the baby's neck. So, let's talk truth. One out of every three babies have their cord around their neck. Most of the time, it's loose and unproblematic. Your baby just spent months snuggling the cord; they are good friends. I once caught a baby who had thrown her cord over her shoulder just before she birthed, as if she was shouldering her purse so she could head out into the world. A skilled provider can catch your baby in such a manner that they roll out with the cord, and it's never tightened around their neck. In the rare incidence that the cord does tighten around the neck, a skilled provider can manage that as well. It usually hasn't been tight for long, and babies are unaffected. Amazing, isn't it?

Take a deep breath. In labor, you fold into yourself, and everything else falls away. Your uterus grabs you and sends you across galaxies to retrieve your baby. With each strong surge of the power that has been sitting within you waiting for this moment, your baby slides through your bones. You give them life; you breathe them into the world with the force of the universe at your back. G-d is in this. You are in this. Nothing like it has come before and nothing like it will come after. Take a deep breath and meet your baby.

The moment mothers first place their babies on their chests, it's as if the whole universe lets go with a sigh of relief. Families melt into each other, mothers are born and you are forever changed.

Chapter Seventeen

What Just Happened?

Postpartum might be one of my favorite topics. It's right up there with sex (hee hee) and talking about my dogs. One reason I like talking about postpartum so much is because it's so under-talked about!

Everyone anticipates the birth, talks about the birth and wants to know the due date and the gender. Then the baby is a week old, and all those birth watchers are gone. Oh, sure, they'll text you at eleven o clock at night wanting to know if you're having contractions, but where are they are at three a.m. when the baby has decided it's time for everyone to be awake?!?! Yes, birth is a big, life-changing event, but it's the beginning of a journey into motherhood for you. Even if it's your ninth child, that new human changes the dynamic of your home and your life.

You have been split open by birth; no matter how or where it happened, your body has undergone a significant change in a fraction of the time it took to build up to that. Think about it; our bodies age over time, gradually over fifty-plus years, but in pregnancy and birth, our bodies stretch, expand, bear a greater weight, squish organs against each other like trying to avoid checking a bag at the airport by cramming everything in a carry-on size and suck nutrients out of our bones, teeth, hair, brain and blood in less than a year. Then what we have created is ejected from our body in a small window of time that seems so long but so short. Just like that, they are separate from us.

I'm a crier. It's just how I handle all emotions. When my babies were no longer inside me, protected by my fluids, muscles and layers of fat, I mourned that change. My baby will never be that close to my heart again. So I cry. This doesn't mean a person with this reaction has postpartum depression. It's a normal adjustment to a big change. If I have a patient who is all sunshine and rainbows during her entire postpartum, I am much more likely to be concerned about underlying postpartum depression than I am with a person who is experiencing a range of emotions. Yes, be overjoyed and swoon over your new baby. Yes, be exhausted and overwhelmed. Yes, be so filled with love for your baby and/or your partner that you cry some more!

Postpartum depression is fairly well-known, thanks to social media. It can pop up any time in your determined postpartum period but is most common within the first five days after birth. In the hours after birth, especially if you birth naturally, your body is floating on oxytocin, that happy hormone. Progesterone, which was elevated during your pregnancy, is also keeping your mood cheery. The lack of sleep, depleted nutrients that were sucked up during your birth and the energy being used to heal can catch up with you and make it hard to stay positive. Around day three to five is when the colostrum in your breasts transitions to milk. In order to make milk, progesterone has to back off so that prolactin can talk to your boobs. The drop in progesterone can cause what most women describe as the "weepies." Just days after your birth, this emotional crash can make you feel helpless.

Birth is huge; it's a major life event (second only to the day you buy your first Chanel bag—just kidding). It's so big that sometimes we forget what happens after the birth. It's hard to comprehend that you will show up in the hours, days, months and years after your birth as a new person. Your whole life has been cracked open, and someone put a baby in it! Your priorities, habits and time management all shift. I once read that babies in the womb grow out toward the world and up toward our hearts. This is so true; your baby lived inside you. Your baby took up space inside your body. Your baby knows the sound of your heartbeat from the inside. They know your movements, your breath, your smell, your hormones and your diet. Your baby has been intimately intertwined in your life.

It took around forty weeks to grow that baby. You followed her movements and tracked his sleep cycles. You protected your baby from harsh words and sharp edges for months, and then in a matter of hours, they are Earthside. I can appreciate that our babies are not truly separate from us really ever, but the transition from physically connected to emotionally, chemically and energetically connected can feel abrupt and intense. It's okay to feel sad about this change, and then ecstatically happy and back again. The transitioning hormones can toy with you. Practice grounding, stay in reality. You are safe; your baby is safe. You are divinely protected.

Remind yourself that you are allowed grace during this change in your life. You can and should ask for help. You have a dinner plate sized wound inside your uterus where your placenta was attached. You have to heal. Wrap up in yourself, your baby and your partner in this period so that you can emerge ready to kick serious ass. I'm serious. Turn off your phone, shut out the world and stay in bed. Fully heal, thank your body over and over again and stare at your baby. I'm right about this—don't test me.

If there is a concern, get help, don't go it alone, recruit the team you built up during your pregnancy, grab other moms, and if you must, do an internet search with caution and a reality filter on. My rule for my clients is on the bed for a week, around the bed for a week and around the house for a week. That's two weeks of staying in your bedroom, resting, napping, eating, drinking and recovering. Followed by a third, fourth, fifth and sixth week or more of keeping life low-key and staying mostly home. If you must go back to work, do so on limited duty. Take it easy.

How many times have I talked about nutrition in this book? Do you think it's important yet? Pregnancy, labor, birth and breastfeeding suck up exorbitant amounts of the nutrients we consume. This doesn't always leave much left for the normal functioning of your body. Take this as a life lesson (in bold because I want you to hear this, highlight it, circle back and write it on your wall): you need to overflow into the world, not sacrifice yourself to it.

This means your life is better lived if you fill your energy and happiness and then overflow into your baby, your partner, your job, your community and your family, rather than serving those other areas first, leaving yourself empty and depleted. Go read it again. You are important, worthy and enough just as you are. Eastern medicine recommends only hot and warm foods during your postpartum period, and I agree. (I know Eastern medicine was waiting for my stamp of approval; you're welcome.) Energetically and physically, mothers have thrown a lot of heat into their labor and birth. During labor, you might have said, "It's so hot in here," while your doula shivered as she held your hand. Heat moves things; it opens, it circulates, it melts the snow off the mountains and awakens our fire! We need that warmth to heal us. Warmth, both in your food and environment, will also help you find your way back into the world after going inside yourself to handle this big thing.

You might feel hungrier than you did in pregnancy—that's normal. You need about 500 more calories a day to support breastmilk, and your body will often let you know this. Have healthy options available in your home, so you aren't tempted to eat junk. Soda is not nourishing! Fast food is not nutrient rich; pre-made frozen food and snacks full of preservatives and dyes are not supportive of a healthy, healing you. Find a good tea and become one of those Zen, goddess-types who eats her vegetables. I believe in you.

Chapter Eighteen

Do I Talk About Vaginas Too Much?

Somewhere in history, a group of medical researchers examined a uterus after a birth (probably more than one, but this is my story) They determined that, on average, a uterus was back to its nonpregnant size and structural integrity (like it's a condo) by six weeks after birth.

Some corporate dude sitting in his shiny office at the insurance company said, "Six weeks is the postpartum period. That's what insurance will cover."

And doctors everywhere said, "It's been six weeks. You're all better now."

While human bodies around the world said, "What timeline?"

I say it now, loudly: expecting anyone to be completely back to pre-pregnancy shape in six weeks is absurd. Many people get hung up on this idea of six weeks. Six weeks is up; it's time to go back to the gym, get back to pre-pregnancy weight, end the mood swings, be full of energy, vibrant, young, hip, busy and back to work. Come on, what's wrong with you?

Screw that. I'm getting mad just writing it. At the time of this writing, I am eighteen months post-birth and to say I feel "back to normal" would not be a whole truth. I feel like I've settled into a new consistency. I feel emotionally more stable, but I'm forever changed by this new person who came with new challenges. As I get older, my belly button might continue to sag until it says hello to my vagina. Who knows what the future holds!

My point is that the postpartum period is defined by the individual who has given birth. For my first two children, right around nine months, I felt ready to expand my life to physical exercise, personal career goals and so on. This also happened to be the time when they made some sort of transition themselves. After my third birth, I felt like I was moving out of a postpartum state when my baby turned a year old. Six weeks is for the birds.

There are a lot more pieces to your postpartum than just the appearance of your uterus, but it is stunning, Darling. Your mental, emotional and hormonal state might need more time. Don't feel pressured to jump right back to your pre-baby life at six weeks. In fact, say good-bye to that life all together. Even your cervix looks different. Before a cervix has dilated for a baby, it looks like a small circular closure. After your cervix opens for your baby (even if you ended up getting a c-section), when your cervix closes, the space in the middle is curved into a smile. Super cool, right? You do not have to have sex, nor do you have to want the same things you did before the baby.

It's also okay to want sex sooner than six weeks, as long as your bleeding has stopped completely, and it feels right to you. Start slow—I mean really slow. Like so much foreplay, you almost cum before any penetration. Even if you were having sex right up until your baby was born, since birth, your body is new. Explore that together, gently, slowly and intimately.

Is feeling "touched out" a thing? YES, yes, yes. It's a thing and it's allowed! Do not feel shame for wanting your partner to touch you less, differently or not at all. Your body just went through a huge thing (have I told you birth is a big deal yet?), and now you are trying to figure out how to move through a new relationship with a tiny, demanding human. If you are breastfeeding, it can feel like your energy is actually pouring out of your breasts, and that doesn't leave you anything to connect physically with additional humans.

That is okay. That is normal and safe. You'll wade through it.

My hope is that your partner is understanding, and the two of you openly communicate and patiently love each other through this period. I will say, with honesty, prior to the birth of my third son, my love language was touch. My partner was fluent in this language. He spoke it often and perfectly. That pregnancy was hard for me. I grieved through a lot of heavy things, and I came out on the other side of that birth and postpartum needing to be loved differently.

My love language changed, and two years later, it hasn't gone back to touch. My sweetheart has been incredible through this transition and taken the time to fight with me to discover this new, amazing version of me, but it was not without a fight. Your partner should be given grace when mistakes are made and communicated with to find new ways to love you. You too must find your voice to share these changes, set boundaries and protect your energy. Sometimes this means showing an unappreciative, disrespectful partner the door. That's okay too. You're here for you now, you're loving yourself now and you're worth it. Fight for it when it deserves your energy; when it doesn't, let it go.

I can't emphasize it enough: be gentle in your postpartum. Yeah, yeah, we know you're amazing, strong and independent, but in this period, your strength lies in your declaration of rest and recovery. Continue to take your supplements, drink water and eat nutrient rich foods.

Because of what I do for work, I know the story of my hairdresser's pregnancies, births, postpartum and breastfeeding experiences. A few days ago, when she was trimming my ends, she said, "I wish someone had told me about the blood postpartum. I had no idea I would bleed that much."

I asked her to elaborate. "How much did you bleed?"

As she ran another strand through her comb, she said, "Just eighteen weeks, but it felt like forever."

I almost jumped out of the chair, but she was near my face with a pair of scissors, so I thought better of it. "Whoa what?" I said, "Sweetie, no, not normal. Where the heck was your team?"

By that I meant her mom, her best friend, her spouse, her doctor and her nurse on the other end of the line. Where was everyone?

"Oh, you know, I just didn't say anything. I was exhausted, but it was kind of embarrassing. I didn't know what to ask."

To be clear, bleeding for eighteen weeks postpartum is not normal and should be assessed by a healthcare provider. You can expect to bleed like a heavy period the first couple of days after birth. Many women use the adult diapers because they catch leaks. You lie down so often, why not dress to match your baby? After this, the bleeding should slow and start to change color, from a bright red to a pink to a brown or brown-red. In the few days after birth, you might lose a clot roughly the size of lime. Losing this clot can cause a small trickle of bleeding that should stop quickly. Repeatedly seeing clots, heavy bleeding, feeling faint, appearing pale or noticing your uterus isn't shrinking or is rising are all cause for concern.

The typical "rule" has been, if you're soaking a pad in an hour or less, that's too much bleeding. When I hemorrhaged, I didn't soak a pad an hour because I spent so much time on the toilet that it just poured out of me in dumps.

When I called the nurse, she said, "Well, if you aren't soaking a pad in less than an hour, you're fine."

You can feel my frustration, right? That was a medical emergency that I ended up in the ER for, by the way.

My point is that you know how much blood seems like too much and when to start asking questions. Don't talk yourself out of taking care of you. Reach out for help, and even if it turns out to be normal or no longer a concern, you can feel heard, validated and worthy of care.

Sometimes, in spite of our best efforts, vaginal lacerations or small abrasions occur. In this case, your care provider can talk through your options. Tears can be small enough that your care provider (if they are knowledgeable in these practices) may offer healing options, like comfrey compress or seaweed. For other tears, many home birth midwives, like myself, are skilled at suturing and can quickly put everything back together at home. However, some midwives don't receive adequate practice in suturing because tears don't happen often in these settings. In that case, your midwife should be humble enough to say, "This is outside of my skill set; we need a pro."

Then they will bring someone in or send you somewhere. This is not an area we trust to just anyone. If your tear is significant, like a complicated second-degree, any third-degree or fourth-degree tear, then an obstetrician is the best option.

Adding to this, currently in Virginia, I cannot carry Lidocaine as a licensed midwife. This means that if I believe a repair will take me more than a few minutes, I'd rather not make anyone suffer unnecessarily, and I send them to an obstetrician who can use numbing meds. I give all moms the choice, of course.

Even if you don't tear, keep your legs together, no lunges, sex or showing off that party trick from your college days where you stick your foot behind your head while taking a shot. Lie down as much as possible to keep fluid from pooling in your vulva region. You can use ice or "padsicles" off and on for the first six hours and then stop. You want fluid with healing nutrients to be able to move in and out of the area; ice will only push fluid away. Herbal compresses of comfrey and calendula, soaked in water, strained, wrapped in something porous like cheese cloth or gauze, then placed between your perineum and your pad can be very helpful. Change the compress each time you go to the bathroom. You can also throw this compress in your tub and do a shallow bath with Epsom salt, although there are times when a bath is not recommended due to infection risk.

The verdict is out on vaginal steaming. Yes, you heard me, vaginal steaming is a thing. I've seen it mentioned in some books, but anecdotally among my midwife friends, there's mixed reviews. If you are unfamiliar, here's a quick run-down: take a pot of water, boil it, add herbs (some recipes even include basil and oregano like you're making spaghetti sauce in your uterus, hey, tu fai tu), place the steaming pot in your toilet so that the brim of the pot is below the brim of the toilet. Next, sit on the toilet and let the steam roll up into your fortress of creation.

Here's my take, is postpartum healing really so difficult that we need to risk scalding? No, not really. On one hand, it could possibly reduce infection with heat. On the other hand, it could increase infection by adding moisture. So, I don't recommend it. The benefit just doesn't outweigh the risk to me, but maybe a graduate student would like to take on this research and please report back if the vagina does, in fact, smell like an Italian restaurant after. Thanks in advance.

An often neglected, but oh so important, topic for postpartum and women's health in general is pelvic floor care. Included in this would specifically be core muscle rehabilitation after pregnancy. The health of these structures starts long before pregnancy. Did anyone else have the parents who echoed "stand up straight," more times than they could count? This was your first introduction to body alignment.

Muscles, fascia, tendons and ligaments make up the pelvic floor in three layers of bone-to-bone connective tissue woven in just the right patterns to support both stability and movement. Your pelvic floor is the shelf that holds up your uterus, bladder and bowels. When you're pregnant, your pelvic floor is the first bed your baby sleeps on. These muscles keep you from peeing yourself all the time. They also hold in and work out your bowel movements. This tissue craves balance; too tight and you get misalignment, inflammation, constipation and a difficult birth. Too loose and your organs fall out if you jump too eagerly out of bed. Having a well taken care of pelvic floor helps with efficient pushing during birth, prevents uterine prolapse, makes sex more pleasurable for both of you (seriously, use your muscle control to tighten down while he's inside you and watch him go crazy) and maintains your good posture. Not to mention it aids with overall function of your entire body by helping keep you in alignment, which helps keep digestion, breathing, circulation and lymphatic movement in an optimal performance state.

In Eastern medicine, your pelvic floor is where you house your sense of safety, your vibrancy and your sexuality (that one is obvious). If you are familiar with acupuncture, then you know about the channels that move through the body. The kidney, spleen, liver, gall bladder, stomach and bladder channels flow through the pelvis and can get gummed up by stagnant chi caused by inflamed tissues or tight or loose muscles that are not at their best.

Do you know your chakras yet? The root chakra sits in this area and is energetically connected to a perineum. The root chakra also holds your sense of trust, belonging and being present. Our bodies hold on to our feelings. Fear, worry, stress, grief and anger end up stored all over our bodies, and they come to the surface as pain, inflammation, poor function, weakness, exhaustion, burn out, overwhelm, disease, acne, difficulty sleeping, hair loss and on and on I could go. Can you imagine how these might also negatively impact pregnancy and childbirth?

Let's say you don't agree with Eastern medicine. The pelvic floor just is, and yours either works or it doesn't. G-d helps those who help themselves. If you never stretch or strengthen the body you were given, that body will not perform the way it was created to. If you never process your very human emotions and traumatic experiences, they will affect the rest of your life, whether you acknowledge it or not. Sugar, ya gotta do the work for you, for your family and for making the most of this life you were given.

Diastasis recti is the separation of your abdominal muscles. What? Your growing uterus is going from approximately seven centimeters to forty centimeters long, and you didn't expect any of your muscles to have to get out of the way? Don't worry, you were made for this (That's it. I'm making a t-shirt that says, "You were made for this." Who has an Etsy shop?). Your muscles separate, and in the months that follow, as you get up, sit down, move, balance, get back into movement and exercise that pleases you, and most of all, carry your baby around using proper posture, your muscles come back together. This might take more conscious effort the more babies you have or the weaker your muscles were coming into pregnancy.

I highly recommend incorporating pelvic floor strengthening and stretching into your exercise routine, and once it is time, start doing core strengthening exercises as well. I also recommend seeking healing and therapy for any difficult emotions that come up in association with birth, sex, penetration, safety, wealth, trust and mindfulness. Your baby is calling you to heal and awaken the strong and flowing person inside you who will raise him.

Chapter Nineteen

D is for "Damn, Girl, Look at You Go"

You grew a PERSON. You were the co-creator of a multi-cellular being! YOU ARE AMAZING! Seriously, stop and acknowledge that. If this book does nothing else for you, may it help you see how truly phenomenal you are. You were once created, cell by cell, bone by bone, organ by organ inside your mother. You were already part of the miracle. Before you got pregnant, before you found someone worth having sex with, you were worthy and incredible. The way your heart beats is enough to leave one awe-stricken.

Your body protected you and your baby. You were divinely protected during your labor journey. Your body opened up to birth your baby. You've birthed the placenta, a whole organ that your body just stitched together like it was bored on a Sunday. A cascade of hormones caused your uterus to contract all the way through labor, birth and into your postpartum to guide you through healing. Of all the breathtaking natural phenomenon I have witnessed, birth is still the most awesome. Not only did your body make your baby, but your body is going to go to the next level and continue to sustain your baby through the first months of life.

Your breasts might have already started leaking, or maybe your partner got a handful and noticed some leakage. If they haven't, not to worry. After your baby is born, once they are placed on your chest—because skin-to-skin with the mother is the BEST place for the baby (I don't have to keep saying that, right?)—you might notice your baby "rooting" or searching around for your breast. Wanna know something cool? Your areola (the skin around your nipple) often gets darker during pregnancy to make it easier for a newborn baby to see! Ha! Your body made a bullseye!

Wait, there's more. You might have also noticed little bumps around and on your areola. Those are pores that secrete fluid to keep your nipple lubricated! Honey, you just get more and more amazing with everything you learn about yourself! When your baby starts opening his mouth and bobbing her head up and down, put a nipple in there! Your baby might start and stop multiple times before really getting the hang of it. Be patient; breastfeeding is like dancing with your baby, and even if you've done it before, this is a new dance partner. Learning to suck, swallow and breathe at the same time takes a little practice.

Just like you, your nipples are unique and special. If your nipples are flat or inverted, you might mention this to your midwife or lactation consultant ahead of time, so you can have a nipple shield available just in case.

During pregnancy and after your baby is born, your body makes colostrum. This is a nutrient-dense liquid that is clear to yellow looking. You don't usually make a lot of colostrum in one sitting, and you aren't meant to. Your baby starts out with a tiny tummy. Your baby should want to breastfeed frequently, and they often act like they haven't eaten in days. I'm a big fan of nursing on demand. From inside your body to the outside world is a HUGE change. The best way to ease this transition is to keep your baby close to you. You are familiar. They know your heartbeat, your breath, your smell; you are safe and warm. Wearing your baby in a wrap or baby carrier can help comfort them and strengthen your core as you practice good posture. In my practice, the mother-baby unit is sacred. You are deeply connected and shall be treated as such.

Three to five days after your birth, the colostrum will transition to milk. This time can be a doozy. To make milk, the hormone prolactin has to increase, which means all that progesterone that got you through pregnancy has to back off. This change can bring on some hard emotional swings. This is what a lot of people describe as being "weepy," which is pretty accurate.

A little crying and identifiable mourning, irritability or anxiety is normal; however, going beyond that into the major doom-and-gloom thoughts of "I am not good," thoughts of suicide, self-harm, harming your baby, not wanting your baby near you, isolating yourself or just feeling straight-up wrong are causes for concern. These are signs of bigger imbalances than the natural flow. Especially if these feelings persist passed the milk transition. There is NO SHAME in these feelings, but you should seek help. You are worth the time and effort to help you get better.

"An ounce of prevention is worth a pound of cure," said Benjamin Franklin. We touched on this earlier, but it's worth revisiting. You know that you will eventually give birth to your baby, so do a little postpartum planning. Gather a team who truly understands your vulnerable state and need to be unburdened, so you can fully recover. Get help with the usual things you do around the house and/or take a stand at your job and get the time off you deserve. Start prepping your significant other and your other children as best you can. They should know you will be singularly focused for a while. Empower them to handle themselves—seriously, this can be good for them and you. Plan to make meals ahead of time and freeze them or have the ingredients in stock. Remember, you need warm, nutrient-dense foods, so plan accordingly. Your energy is needed for establishing breastfeeding and healing. I mean it, the rest of the world can wait; you have more important things to tend to.

One question I get regularly is "Are my boobs too small to make enough milk?"

No, no, a thousand times no. The size of your breasts has nothing to do with the amount of milk you produce. Previous breast surgeries might affect breastfeeding depending on the type of surgery and how it went. I am an A-cup, at most, and I spent a good portion of my life wishing they were bigger. I have fully appreciated my breasts in two areas of my life. The first being breastfeeding, because they have always seemed to rise to the occasion, even if they needed some help initially. The second is while running down my stairs, which I didn't completely grasp until my breasts tripled in size during my third pregnancy, and I was forced to cradle them every time I lightly jogged anywhere. They have now returned to their original size, and I can skip-to-my-loo all the live-long day! My point is, of all the things that affect milk supply, breast size is not one of them.

This is the time for you and your baby; continue to set boundaries. Anyone who visits can do a chore and keep the visit short. They don't need to hold your baby. Your baby is an extension of you. If you wouldn't let all those people touch you, why are they touching your baby? People can F right off, as far as I'm concerned. You have just passed an entire human through your bones, Queen. You are worthy of rest.

I'm not intentionally ignoring formula-fed babies. I subscribe to the breast-is-best belief and encourage mothers to try. If breastfeeding is not possible in spite of your best efforts, there are some good quality formulas on the market. Do your research and find the formula you trust the most.

Have you heard of tongue ties? They are all the rage this season. Either more babies have tongue ties or practitioners have just gotten better at recognizing them. I was educated on tongue ties by a pediatric dentist years ago, but I'm still meeting pediatricians who claim they don't exist! I have a close frustration with tongue ties because I entered the postpartum of my last baby thinking, "I've got this. I've done this before. Breastfeeding is my favorite part!"

I got a week into breastfeeding, and my nipples were so sore, I couldn't wear shirts! My supply was not adequate, and my sweet baby wasn't gaining weight as we'd expected. I called three specialists, and they all made the same statements:

"It's probably your latch."

"Try pumping instead."

"For a small fee of $399, I can do an assessment in my office."

It was infuriating! We had a problem. I committed every fiber of my being and every ounce of brain power I had left after an exhausting pregnancy to solve this problem. I took the supplements, ate the lactation cookies, cereal and granola bars. I even tried this powdered supplement that supposedly helps improve milk supply, but the advertisement did not say "tastes like dirt." I couldn't count ounces while I was gagging, so maybe it worked. I was measuring my value in ounces every day! I power pumped. I pumped every hour. I nursed and then pumped. I cried through the pain every time he latched. My midwife found a donor to supply breast milk to support my baby's weight gain while I worked on my own supply. I felt worthless.

I actually talked to my boobs. "Come on, girls, half an ounce more, just . . . no, don't quit, just a little more. Please, what do you want from me?!?!?"

I saw my doctor and paid hundreds of dollars to get lab work done only to hear, "According to your labs, your hormones are fantastic. You should be making plenty of milk. I can't explain it."

A month of 24/7 obsessing about my boobs and the health of my baby went by. A midwife mentor of mine suggested I call a lactation consultant we both knew. I did. I described what was going on through tear-soaked words.

"Dev, it sounds like he has a tongue tie," she said, intuitively over the phone.

I booked an appointment with a pediatric dentist for an assessment. They told me they would assess him, but my insurance doesn't cover any of it. I didn't care. I would have given anything to get my blissful breastfeeding experience. At the assessment, the dentist identified a posterior tie. We scheduled a revision.

The revision took three minutes, no joke. I didn't notice a difference right away, which was heartbreaking. "My nipples are going to hurt forever!" I told my baby's dad.

For the next two weeks, each day got a little better. The first day I caught two ounces from the breast my baby was not attached to, I cried and sent a picture of it to anyone who had heard me talk about my boobs for the last six weeks (which was all I talked about, to anyone I came across).

The lady at my local coffee shop had even started asking me about my nipples. Can you imagine?

Her: "Hi, how are you?"

Me: (bursting into tears) "I'm failing as a mother because I can't make enough milk, and I don't know why. My nipples feel like they're being cut off if my shirt even brushes up against them. How are you?"

It was a journey. Eighteen months later, he's still snuggling in to nurse, and I have even been blessed enough to be able to donate milk to other babies! My point in sharing this is to first explain that sometimes we really do have to throw our whole selves at a problem, and it really can be worth it. My second point is to drive home my belief in the impact of tongue ties. Babies need their whole tongue to nurse efficiently. When they can't use their whole tongue, they get tired faster and fall asleep before draining the entire breast, thus creating a lack of demand and a lower supply. This restricted movement also causes them to compensate with other muscles, which leads to excessive tension in their jaw muscles. This can lead to poor posture, tension headaches and speech problems as they get older. The entire body is connected, and one malfunctioning movement pattern can throw off the rest of the system. If you ever get the chance find an ultrasound of a baby nursing on the internet, it is super cool to watch and provides a good visual of just how much they need their whole tongue.

Your baby should get a head-to-toe inspection within the hours after birth, and whoever does this should be trained in identifying tongue ties or humble enough to say this baby needs another set of eyes. If you aren't sure or if breastfeeding isn't going well, seek a tie specialist to evaluate your baby as one of the steps in problem solving. Speech pathologists and pediatric dentists are currently the experts I refer to.

Chapter Twenty
Hello, Baby

There's nothing in the world like staring at a baby. All their tiny parts, all their bundled-up potential, their vulnerable, authentic innocence—they melt our hearts. We watch them hit milestones and ache as they grow more and more into the world. Every mark, noise, bump, scratch, sniffle, cough and cry sends us into a spiral of concern and internet searches. You are the perfect mother for your baby. Everything your baby needs is you.

When babies first enter the world, they are, well, goopy. They are wet with amniotic fluid, maybe spotted with blood and sometimes coated in a white frosting-like substance called vernix. Don't bathe your baby for at least a week. You can wipe up obvious smears of blood or poop, but otherwise, let their skin be. Vernix is a white layer of goo that coats your baby in the uterus. If you were to sit in water for nine months, you'd look like a raisin. Vernix acts as a thick layer of lotion to protect your baby during prolonged exposure to amniotic fluid. The longer your baby stays inside, the less vernix they will be born with. You might still find it in the creases of their thigh and armpits—just leave it. The vernix will be absorbed or naturally rub off over the next day.

Now for the routine care part. I am referred to as a traditional midwife. The term conventional is often used to describe obstetrical care, hospital care or nurse midwife care. This is difficult for me because the definitions make the care seem so different from each other. Traditional sounds old and hippie, while conventional is the care accepted by the general public. This is not the world I live in. I have a clinic, a practice, a license, practice documents, faxing and filing systems, the ability to order and draw labs, and I document and communicate in medical terms. For my clients' hour-long visits, discussions of various options and respect for their personal preferences is the norm. I often forget that there are people who don't know home birth is an option or that they have the ability to decline practitioner recommendations. I'll use these terms here, but to be clear, they aren't adequate.

In conventional medicine, the routine immediately after birth is babies receive a hepatitis B vaccination, a vitamin K injection and antibiotic eye ointment. We'll talk through this a little. The hepatitis B virus was first discovered as a disease-causing virus in 1967 by medical anthropologist Baruch Blumberg. That's not super relevant to this book, but it feels right to give him credit as if winning a Nobel Prize isn't credit enough. It moved quickly (as viruses go) to isolation, vaccine development and FDA approval in 1981. Did you track that? From 1967 to 1981, a snail's pace compared to the recent COVID-19 shutdowns to vaccination release.

In its early years, the vaccine was only recommended for members of high-risk status, such as refugees from countries with high hepatitis numbers, individuals with risqué sexual behaviors like multiple unprotected partners, and intravenous drug users. Ten years later, the FDA changed their tune and decided everyone everywhere needed this vaccine. To be clear, your baby can only get hepatitis B if you, the mother, have hepatitis B. In 1997, it was implemented that childcare facilities had to require the hepatitis B vaccine because three-year-olds are obviously swapping dirty needles in the back of storytime. This is why vaccination started at birth and progressed through the early years in a multiple shot routine.

"My doctor gives me attitude if I decline a vaccine."

Listen, declining or doing any or all vaccines is your right, but your doctor has a different perspective than you do. Respect their stance and background while making your own choices. Doctors can be audited and reprimanded for not "providing quality care" if patients don't get vaccinated. This is nonsense, I know. While we would like all our doctors to push back against this and get paid for care that is respectful of our choices, that's not the way things are— yet. So go easy on your doctor and find one you like who respects your decision despite the people at the big tables breathing down their necks.

Vitamin K is just that—a vitamin made by nature and discovered by a German guy (I'm only assuming because the 'K' stands for Koagulation, which is German). Vitamin K is fat-soluble, meaning it is stored in our fat, versus water-soluble like vitamin C, which we urinate out on a regular basis. Vitamin K molecules are hefty and therefore don't pass through the placenta or into breast milk. Babies are naturally born with "vitamin K deficiency." Using the word deficiency makes this sound like a problem, but it actually appears to be by design, like on purpose, like whoever or whatever is responsible for this had a reason upon development.

We get vitamin K from two places: dark leafy greens and our own gut. Babies aren't born eating kale, and their guts need some priming first. This happens over time for breast-fed babies, which is why their risk decreases as time goes on. There are some good, quality formulas on the market, many of which contain vitamin K for your baby.

Vitamin K is one factor in our blood that helps with clotting. Vitamin K deficiency bleeding is when a baby bleeds, internally or externally, without the ability to clot. Granted, babies are born with platelets (another clotting factor that works differently), so they aren't totally unprotected here. Vitamin K deficiency bleeding is rare, and the risk increases with the use of certain medications used by the mother, like anticoagulants and certain seizure meds.

There are three options for vitamin K administration after birth: decline all together, injection in the thigh with a tiny needle or oral administration. You need to know there is no such thing as a completely preservative-free vitamin K medication. Preservatives are well known for causing other problems including breathing complications and metabolism dysfunction.

Whether or not you decide on vitamin K supplementation for your baby might be influenced by whether or not you decide to have your baby circumcised. If you want to have your son circumcised, some practitioners require vitamin K administration. Some will only accept an injected vitamin K; others will accept the oral dose.

I'm not going to make any "do it" or "don't do it" statements here, because that's not my job. In fact, I hope this entire book is letting you know that you have a choice, and you deserve to have that choice respected. My goal is to present information and let you choose. Again, the choices are personal to you and your family. If this basic information is not adequate, I encourage you to research and seek a second opinion.

It is my general recommendation that families wait until at least a week post-birth to get their baby circumcises. Babies are working very hard to do a lot of transitioning. Why add the stress of pain and healing on to that? In addition, their risk of vitamin K deficiency bleeding goes down after the first seven days. So maybe the Jews were on to something when they circumcised on the eighth day . . . maybe I'm biased.

Erythromycin is currently the antibiotic of choice routinely administered as a drop into the newborn's eyes after birth. If a mother is positive for gonorrhea when her baby passes through her vagina, there's a risk that a newborn will develop an infection of the eye(s) that can lead to blindness. Many women are routinely tested for chlamydia and gonorrhea in early pregnancy. Some women are also tested if they show up to the hospital in labor. Individuals at risk would be those who have changed sexual partners since their last STD screening and people with multiple sexual partners.

I want you to be able to enjoy your baby and practice breastfeeding, but let's talk about just two more routine care things. First is the newborn screen, which used to be called the PKU because it started out being a test just for phenylketonuria (PKU). Today this test includes: phenylketonuria, hypothyroidism, cystic fibrosis, sickles cell anemia, galactosemia, maple syrup urine disease, homocystinuria, biotinidase deficiency, congenital adrenal hyperplasia, medium chain acyl-CoA dehydrogenase deficiency (MCAD), tyrosinemia, citrullinemia, beta thalassemia, hemoglobin SC disease, severe combined immunodeficiency, Pompe disease, mucopolysaccharidosis, spinal muscle atrophy, X-linked adrenoleukodystrophy and the list goes on. Please don't make me keep going.

You can see that these sound pretty serious. They are. These conditions can be life-threatening or cause permanent damage if they are left untreated. This is why it became recommended that all states require the newborn screen. Each state varies on the exact requirements, but in general, they are pretty close.

This test usually takes place at your 24-hour postpartum visit for an out-of-hospital birth or before you leave the hospital if you birthed there. Have you ever had your finger poked for a blood test? The needle used is in a plastic case, and it shoots out when it is pressed against your finger. This is a lancet, and the same device is used on your newborn's heel. It's a tiny needle, and the device has a controlled depth. Drops of blood are collected onto a card. All the circles on the card have to be filled and saturated, so this can take some time. Most babies fuss a little when they are poked and then get a little perturbed while their foot is being held, but it doesn't seem to bother them much overall. I say this based on the newborns that I test, and I believe the underwhelming reaction I get from newborns is because they are nestled in their mother's arms or contently nursing while I play with their foot. Other practices might not do it this way.

Once the blood is collected and dried on the card, the card is filled out with the mother's name, the baby's name and information about the baby's weight, birth date and time, whether or not the mother was adopted and the care provider's information. It's mailed to an official state lab and results are sent back to the provider. Depending on the state, an abnormal result might prompt a call to the care provider, instructing them to get immediate care for the newborn. Some of my clients have concerns that the blood being sent to the state is also being used for genetic experiments, storing DNA information on their baby or something not in line with their ethics. I don't have evidence of these practices.

There is also some question as to whether mandating a test is ethical, and as you know, your girl is all about choice. I can't speak to the action of all states if you decline this test. I do know some states send a letter basically shaming the parents and the care provider when the test is not performed. Besides this written slap on the wrist, there aren't other consequences. However, the same state telling you to take this test is also in charge or your care provider's credentialing, and they might threaten that. It is my personal opinion that, for this particular routine care, the benefits do outweigh the risks, but my opinion might not mean jack to you, and that's okay.

Two more tests to go, then I'll leave you alone to snuggle and stare at your baby. The hearing screen is pretty simple. There are two types of testing options. The most common is the Otoacoustic Emissions (OAE) screening. A small device is placed in your baby's ear, a sound is sent into the ear and then whether or not that sound is echoed back is measured. The second option uses a microphone device and sticker electrodes on the baby's head to measure automated auditory brainstem response (AABR). If no sound echoes back, it's an indication that the baby was born with hearing loss and further assessment is recommended. The sooner hearing loss is detected, the sooner intervention can take place. If a hearing loss diagnosis is missed, developmental delays can take place.

You know what they did before these fancy machines were invented? Parents paid attention to their babies and noticed if their babies did not respond to sound. Most babies will turn toward noise, show some sort of recognition of sound like opening their eyes, moving their eyebrows, mouth or eyes, jumping in a startle reaction or trying to look at the noise. If these responses are lacking, the baby might not be able to hear. The sound sent out by the machine does not pose a significant risk to damaging tissues in the ear and the test is usually quick. A minimally invasive process overall. Not all practices own these expensive machines. They will likely recommend where you can go to get it.

The last routine test is the CCHD screen. This stands for critical congenital heart defects. The test involves placing a pulse oximeter on your baby's right hand and right foot and assessing the numbers given. The percentages are expected to be above 95 percent and a less than 3 percent difference between the hand and foot. This screening is often done when your baby is around twenty-four hours old, although I'm aware of some practitioners who do this an hour or so after birth and then repeat it at twenty-four hours. A number less than 95 percent or greater difference than 3 percent indicate a heart complication and further assessment is necessary to determine which heart complication is at play.

The basis of all these tests is early detection. These tests can lead to identifying life-threatening conditions that can be treated with early intervention. Most of the babies in my care sleep or nurse right through these screenings and are completely unbothered. While these screenings can be valuable, they should still be done in a respectful way.

In my practice, I step out of the room (but still within ear shot) and leave the mother to bond with her baby after the birth. This time is important. Moms are given the opportunity to recollect themselves mentally and emotionally after they just traveled through galaxies to retrieve their baby. Fathers/partners get to breathe in this moment—they just held their breath in anticipation for three hours. I encourage families to let go of all the stress from the anticipation they have carried until the birth of their baby. Fifteen minutes later, I pop back in to say, "How is everyone doing?"

I listen to the baby with my stethoscope and check on the mother's bleeding. Then I leave again. It could be two hours before I ask the mother if she's ready for me to move her baby off of her and do a head-to-toe examination of her baby. The newborn screen and CCHD are done at about twenty-four hours after birth, and the hearing screen is recommended sometime in the first three months.

If there is nothing immediately wrong, there's no reason to interrupt that essential bonding between babies and their person.

Other things you might not have known you were getting when you asked for a baby:

Meconium is poop that your baby was making while they were practicing interpretive dance with your belly button. Meconium is black, sticky and a good sign that your baby's colon and rectum are in good working order. Sometimes babies poop before they are born. This is diluted by the amniotic fluid and usually not a concern. On the rare occasion a baby aspirates meconium in utero, normally their bodies will process this out. Occasionally they need a little extra help inflating their lungs or fighting an infection.

The umbilical cord might smell. Not to worry, keep it dry and clean. It will fall off and leave a moist looking area that will dry and heal on its own.

Your baby might sound congested. Try to remember they are coming from a water environment. Some of the water and goop from birth might have gotten sucked up their nose or swallowed. More often than not, they process that out. Enjoy the cute little whistle when they breath. If they sound congested for an extended period, sneeze frequently, have snot or booger build up or develop a fever, you can squirt some breast milk up their nose or use the sterile saline sprays from your local pharmacy. Breastmilk is a natural antibiotic, and the fluid will loosen mucus to help it come out. Saline solution is alkaline that creates an environment less than desirable for bacteria and viruses, and the fluid also loosens mucus.

Colic is said to be excessive crying without a cause, but as time goes on, we're learning that this "uncontrollable" crying is likely due to digestive upset. This can be caused by a number of things. If your baby is breastfed, they might be sensitive to a food you're eating. Common problematic foods include eggs, broccoli, garlic, coffee, soda, other cruciferous vegetables, dairy, gluten, corn, onion and soy products. Cut any or all of these out of your diet for thirty days and see if things improve. It's difficult to identify the exact food; it can take trial and error. Your baby could also grow out of this food sensitivity, so you might be able to work the food back into your diet, especially as they nurse less. Your baby might never outgrow this sensitivity, and that food just won't be part of their life. Tummy massage, leg movements and a practitioner-approved probiotic for baby can also be helpful solutions.

Diaper rash, baby acne and cradle cap are normal baby things. Diaper rash is usually easily managed by letting your baby air-out by going diaper free for periods of time and with a simple diaper rash cream, the more hippie the better. Don't use corn starch or baby powder.

Baby acne is also normal—don't pop it. You can rub a little breastmilk on it or leave it alone completely. Their skin is just adjusting. Pay attention to detergents, soaps, wipes, lotions and other things coming into contact with your baby's skin. These can cause rashes, acne, redness or eczema. Cradle cap, otherwise known as baby dandruff, is just their scalp shedding. A gentle, silicone cradle cap brush can be helpful for clearing it up but also not necessary. It's not a concern, doesn't bother your baby and doing anything about it is mostly for appearances. Do not pick at it.

Arriving alongside your precious bundle is a custom delivery of sleep deprivation, adult diapers and spit-up on every shirt you want to wear. I'll be upfront with you, sleep training is not in this book, not because I'm not familiar with the different methods but because, in my experience as a mom and care provider, babies who are catered to in their early years thrive more later on. I encourage moms to land somewhere between attachment parenting and no parenting.

Our babies need the safety and security the familiarity of their family offers. Balancing this with Mom's ability to get sleep, self-care, work or just a moment of her body to herself is the struggle of parenting. It is also possible. Stay present, treasure and soak in every moment. The moment your baby falls asleep holding your breast. The moment you get to sink into a warm bath all by yourself. Even the moment when your baby is crying, and you are the only one who can calm their distress.

I know it's cliché, but we are not our baby's everything forever. Hold every moment while you have it, and then let it go to embrace the next good thing.

Chapter Twenty-one
You Are What You Think

I considered sharing birth stories throughout this book, but the truth is, I have no desire to fluff you up with stories of moms breathing through labor then birthing their babies out with an orgasm and a glass of wine. Sure, I've seen it; it's possible. I've watched women cuss, scream, breathe, pant, grunt, pray, bite, throw things, walk, roll, dance, punch and sing their babies out. Every mom, baby, family and birth is unique. Whatever story you and your baby write is beautiful. The moans of your birth song are the miracle of humankind in your custom melody.

The birth story that had the greatest impact on me happened when I was attending births on the US/Mexico border. I was more exhausted than I have ever been in my life. I often went days with no more than twenty-minute power naps because the babies just kept coming. One night, a seventeen-year-old girl showed up on the birth center front porch. She had only been in for two prenatal visits her entire pregnancy. That was not new; many of the families we cared for could only make the trip over the border a few times during their pregnancies. Immigration policy is a debate for another book. I was tasked with keeping mothers and babies alive. This was my only focus.

She rang the obnoxiously loud doorbell meant to wake everyone up. Three of us met her at the door. We pushed open the old screen door and invited her in. She was followed by her mother. Between contractions, we led her down the hall into a room with a bed where she could birth. Her labor was long and hard. She worked through one contraction after another into the morning and on into that night. During more intense moments of transition, exhaustion and frustration, we learned this pregnancy was the result of rape by her uncle. She cried, her mom cried and we cried. Coming to our birth center in the darkness of night was more than taking a trip to meet her baby; it was an escape. She was fleeing something heavier than all of us. Her labor held the pain and fear of her abuse, exploitation, persecution, family ridicule and despair.

I will never forget her screams. She said things like, "Please, kill me! Make it stop. Just kill me now!"

It was heartbreaking. The kind of thing that makes you want to pack up and decide being a midwife is not for you.

Her birth team consulted and asked her if she would be more comfortable in a hospital where she could get pain medication. She begged us not to send her where a man might touch her body again. I put her face in my hands, locked my green eyes on her brown ones and said, "You are safe. This is your body."

She wrapped her arms around me and squeezed as the next contraction took her. She screamed. I wished so badly I could hold her pain for her. I cried into her hair. We melted together as I held her up.

A midwife on our team said, "I see a head."

I let out my breath. Finally, we were close.

At 4:44 in the morning, her small, covered in goop and wailing baby rested in the midwife's arms.

I locked eyes with the midwife and put up my finger, asking her to wait. I moved the mother's sweaty head off my chest and brushed back her black hair.

"Your baby is here. Are you ready?" I held intense eye contact and waited for her to tell me she was ready to meet her baby.

"I can't," she whimpered. I knew what she meant. We've all come to that place. When we just can't be the mom. We just can't greet our children with a smile—not again, not today.

"You can. You can do anything. You are worthy," I said softly to her in Spanish.

She took a couple more breaths, still holding me tightly. Her baby wiggled and let out small yells. After one long exhale, she looked up at me. "Something else is there!"

I kept my voice soft. "Si, esa es la placenta." I told her it was okay, and another member of our team held a bowl under her to catch it.

Now that she was no longer pregnant, a wave swept over her, and the color in her face had a pink hue. She shuffled her feet back and then turned. She saw her baby and burst into loud cries.

"A boy!" she yelled. "A boy to save us! A strong boy! My boy! My boy! My boy!" She scooped him into her arms like she had known him for centuries. She noticed little else for the next day. We tucked her into bed and talked at length, but she never took her eyes off her baby. She named him Arman, for hope.

If you're wondering, she did return for some postpartum care but not much. Her mother arranged for her to move in with her aunt who was living in the United States. We directed them toward the office they would need to navigate immigration paperwork. I like to believe Arman brought her the hope Mom needed and showed her the strength she already had.

I have witnessed the colossal strength of women time and time again. This is why I am often insulted and frustrated when I watch women stifle themselves for the sake of fragile egos and people pleasing. Your story doesn't have to look like this teenage girl's to be a demonstration of strength. Just greeting the world, navigating choices, holding together relationships, running a household, steering a career, and getting everyone to sports events, church and birthday parties less than fifteen minutes late takes strength. Healing from trauma and working through all the ways we are insecure and human takes strength. Wading through the muck of persecution, discrimination, harassment, assault, aggression and microaggressions chipping away at you is strength.

You are capable of eating well, exercising and taking care of your body for an optimal pregnancy. You are capable of making choices about your healthcare and your birth experience. Damn, Girl, you are even able to take a birth experience that didn't go exactly as planned and view it in a way that provides you growth, peace and maybe the drive to make the world a better place. I have to believe I am here to be more than a victim, more than a bystander to my own life.

You enter your labor to birth an entirely new person into the world, and you become a new person in this process. The pain of birth has a purpose and so does the pain of growth. As we learn to set boundaries, we process the guilt of not performing the way others say we should. As we change careers, locations, partners, lifestyles and habits, we feel the discomfort of starting something new. We don't know as much—we must find another way, struggle through the trauma responses and experience the growing pains.

I hear you. There's an excuse. There's a reason that you are really attached to. I can't talk you out of it. I can't do the work for you. I have been married twice and divorced twice. I have a sexual violence history, divorced parents and daddy issues. I nearly died from a hemorrhage after an abortion, had an unexplained emergency C-section at nineteen years old, attempted suicide, and if you really wanna go there, my people were enslaved, banished, persecuted and murdered for hundreds of years across multiple countries. I could wallow in that history. I could also demand that G-d never make anything hard for me again, because I've been through enough, but that's not what I'm here for. I'm here to face hard things, then take those experiences and make something good to put back into the world. Get sick of your own excuses. Get tired of letting other people hold your power. Your parents' behavior, your boss's attitude, your rapist's actions are not on you. You are bigger and more of a badass than they could ever imagine! Cry it out, Mama, then go change your shirt (seriously, you leaked through that one already) and go get everything you want.

With love,

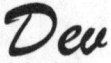

131

Key Terms

ABO: The various blood types. A, AB, and O.

AF: As fuck. Millennial slang meaning a lot or a fuck ton.

anterior: An anatomical direction referring to the front of the body.

Braxton Hicks: Contractions that do not progress to birth.

CBC: Complete Blood Count.

chorioamnionitis: An infection of the amniotic fluid and the membranes around it.

g-spot: A pressure point inside the vagina that feels pleasurable when pressure is applied to it.

GBS: Group B Streptococcus.

lotus birth: During birth and throughout the postpartum, the umbilical cord is not cut. Instead, it dries and falls off, keeping the baby attached to the placenta until it falls off naturally.

membranes: In this book, membranes refer to the "bag" holding the "water" (amniotic fluid) in which the baby is growing in utero. Membranes are what break or rupture at some point during birth or shortly after.

meningitis: An infection that causes inflammation of the membranes around the spinal cord and brain. This can have life-long effects and may be caused by bacteria or a virus.

missionary: Sexual position traditionally known as the man on top.

Mofo: Shorthand for mother fucker.

monogamous: A style of relationship that involves one person being in a relationship with only one other person.

placenta: The accessory organ that develops with pregnancy to transport nutrients, waste and oxygen between the mother and baby.

polyamorous: The word translates as "many loves" and applies when someone has multiple lovers or romantic relationships at the same time with everyone's knowledge and consent.

prodromal: Also known as false labor, a pattern of contractions that does not progress to active labor.

self-exploration: Also known as masturbation but not limited to penetration of the vagina. Can include touching, thinking or using assistive devices to cause sexual pleasure for oneself.

ta-day: Slang for "today."

UTI: Urinary Tract Infection. A build-up of bacteria in the tube running from the bladder to the outside world.

References

American Academy of Audiology. https://www.audiology.org/consumers-and-patients/children-and-hearing-loss/newborn-hearing-screening/, 2022

Centers For Disease Control and Prevention. https://www.cdc.gov/ncbddd/heartdefects/hcp.html, 2022

Coad, Jane and Melvyn Dunstall. Anatomy and Physiology for Midwives (3rd ed.). Churchill Livingstone, Elsevier, London, UK, 2011.

Chapman, Vicky and Cathy Charles. The Midwife's Labour and Birth Handbook (4th ed). John Wiley and Sons LTD, Chichester, West Sussex, UK, 2018.

Florida Healthy Kids Corporation. www.healthykids.org, 2023.

Frye, Anne. Holistic Midwifery, A Comprehensive Textbook for Midwives in Homebirth Practice, Vol. 1: Care During Pregnancy. Labrys Press, Portland, OR, 2013.

Frye, Anne. Holistic Midwifery, A Comprehensive Textbook for Midwives in Homebirth Practice, Vol. II: Care During Labor and Birth. Labrys Press, Portland, OR, 2013.

Gruenberg, Bonnie. Birth Emergency Skills Training. Birth Muse Press, Duncannon, PA, 2008.

Johnson, Ruth and Wendy Taylor. Skills for Midwifery Practice (4th ed). Churchill Livingstone, Elsevier, London, UK, 2016.

King, Tekoa, Mary Brucker, Jan Kriebs, Jenifer Fahey, and Carolyn Gegor (2014). Varney's Midwifery (5th ed). Jones and Bartlett Learning, Burlington, MA, 2014

Manning, Loretta and Sylvia Rayfield. Pharmacology Made Insanely Easy (5th ed.). I CAN Publishing Inc., Duluth, GA, 2017.

Marshall, Jane and Maureen Raynor. Myles Textbook for Midwives (16th ed). Churchill Livingstone, Elsevier, London, UK, 2014.

Moore, Keith, T.V.N. Persaud, and Mark Torchia. Before We were Born: Essentials of Embryology and Birth Defects (9th ed.) Churchill Livingstone, Elsevier, London, UK, 2015.

Public Health England. https://www.gov.uk/government/news/screening-pregnant-women-for-gbs-not-recommended, 2017

Thomas, Paul and Jennifer Margulis. The Vaccine Friendly Plan. Penguin Random House LLC, New York, 2016.

The VBAC Link. How to Really Understand the Risk for Uterine Rupture. https://www.thevbaclink.com/uterine-rupture/, 2023.

WebMD LLC. What are the Risks of a C-Section? https://www.webmd.com/baby/risks-of-a-c-section, 2023.

Cunningham, F. Gary, Kenneth Leveno, Steven Bloom, Catherine Spong, Jodi Dashe, Barbara Hoffman, Brian Casey, and Jeanne Sheffield. Williams Obstetrics (24th ed). McGraw Hill Education, New York, NY, 2014.

Acknowledgements

I am overflowing with gratitude as I sit down to write the last piece of this book. I will start by thanking the midwives I've encountered along the way.

Sandhano was the first midwife to teach me to trust myself and my body. Thank you for catching my second baby and for suggesting that I become a midwife. You are wise beyond comparison, and you changed my whole life.

Janelle, my mentor and friend, you gave me the confidence to dive into owning my own practice. You were an incredible teacher and continue to be my treasured friend.

Lorri, there are no words to describe what a phenomenal and inspiration woman you are. I could spend a decade as your apprentice and still not know everything you know. Thank you for your guidance and for throwing me into the deep end on occasion; that's where I really learned.

Thank you, Hayley Swedelius. From the moment we met at the first birth I ever attended until today, you've been my rock in hard times and there to celebrate all my wins. You get me, and it's so incredibly powerful to feel fully seen and fully loved. I hope I am as good to you as you are to me. Thank you for existing.

Thank you, thank you, thank you, Jessica Baynes. You have made me a better human. Your deep respect and love for every person you meet is unparalleled and so easy to see. You truly embody Jesus in all that you do. Now I'm going to start crying, so moving on . . .

Forever would not be enough time to show gratitude for my partner John. I am so glad we found each other. You've given me more love, appreciation, respect, romance and laughter than I could ever imagine. Thank you for being the man you are.

A huge thank you to my kids for cheering me on, being patient when I needed to work on my book and always being up for a new, fun adventure. I love you all with my whole heart.

Thank you to my mom who has opened her heart and mind to her rebel daughter's wild ways. I am the Earth shaker you raised me to be. Thank you for not coddling me or making excuses for me. You empowered me to never settle and to chase all my dreams. In case you ever wonder, you have been everything I needed in a mom and more. I love you.

I don't know if it makes sense to write a thank you to someone who isn't here anymore, but thank you, Dad, for all the ways you were trying to be everything to everyone and how that taught me to embrace the big heart you gave me while loving myself like you did. Thank you for our last year together, for protecting me in every way you could. I love you, Dad. Rest in peace.

I could say thank you a million times to the team that made this book possible. To my editor, Dawn, thank you for all your guidance, feedback and for making parts of my book not sound like I was drunk when I wrote them (I wasn't for the record). This book would not have happened without you.

To the photographer who created the cover photo, Whitney. The moment I sat across from you in that coffee shop and said, "I'm thinking two speculums talking."

And you responded, "In bed?"

I knew we were destined to work together. Our pillow-talking speculums are a feat only you could accomplish. Thank you for sharing your talent.

Thank you, Noelle, the best makeup artist on the East Coast. The confidence boost you have given me by showing me how to care for and enhance my face is priceless. Not only are your makeup skills personalized to perfection, but your sense of humor is magnetic!

I have felt so loved and supported throughout the entire process of writing this book. Thank you to Chemerre, the creator and owner of the coffee shop where I wrote this book and enjoyed many cups of coffee.

Thank you to one of the first to read my book, Marie Baker, for your ever-honest friendship and feedback.

Thank you, Hashem, for blessing me beyond measure.

About the Author

Dev Honey is a licensed midwife and mother of four. After her own emergency C-section and first home vaginal birth after c-section, Dev was driven to support other laboring parents. She traveled across the U.S. and to foreign soil to gain experience and has been called to attend births on the U.S.-Mexico border at a high-volume birth center. Dev owns Birds and Bees Midwifery, LLC, a maternity care practice where she cares for hundreds of pregnant people and assists other midwives build their practices.

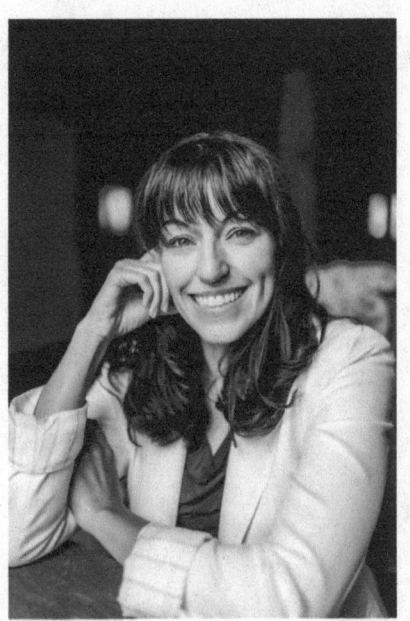